W9-BXN-141

Philosophic
Inquiry
in Nursing

To Rozella Schlotfeldt

Philosophic Inquiry in Nursing

*

Edited By
June F. Kikuchi
Helen Simmons

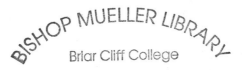
BISHOP MUELLER LIBRARY
Briar Cliff College
SIOUX CITY, IA 51104

SAGE Publications
International Educational and Professional Publisher
Newbury Park   London   New Delhi

Copyright © 1992 by Sage Publications, Inc.

All rights reserved. No part of this book may be reproduced or utilized in any form or by any means, electronic or mechanical, including photocopying, recording, or by any information storage and retrieval system, without permission in writing from the publisher.

RT
84.5
.P5
1992

For information address:

SAGE Publications, Inc.
2455 Teller Road
Newbury Park, California 91320

SAGE Publications Ltd.
6 Bonhill Street
London EC2A 4PU
United Kingdom

SAGE Publications India Pvt. Ltd.
M-32 Market
Greater Kailash I
New Delhi 110 048 India

Printed in the United States of America

Library of Congress Cataloging-in-Publication Data

Main entry under title:
Philosophic inquiry in nursing / edited by June F. Kikuchi, Helen
   Simmons.
         p.   cm.
   Includes bibliographical references and index.
   ISBN 0-8039-4460-8 (cl).   — ISBN 0-8039-4461-6 (pb)
   1. Nursing—Philosophy—Congresses. 2. Nursing—Research—
Methodology—Congresses.   I. Kikuchi, June F. II. Simmons, Helen,
1927-
[DNLM: 1. Philosophy, Nursing.   WY 86 P568]
610.73'01—dc20   91-42002

92 93 94 95   10 9 8 7 6 5 4 3 2 1

Sage Production Editor: Diane S. Foster

4792983

Contents

✳

Acknowledgments

✳

We are indebted to the contributing authors of this volume. It is primarily by virtue of their pioneering spirit in their willingness to disclose their reflections in a virtually unexplored territory—philosophic inquiry in nursing—that this collection of essays came to be.

We wish to express our gratitude to those graduate nursing students at the University of Alberta whose desire and commitment to philosophize about their world strengthened our resolve to establish the Institute for Philosophical Nursing Research. In the name of that Institiute, we wish to express our appreciation to all those who have contributed to the production of this volume in various ways: the Winspear Foundation and the University of Alberta for their financial support; Tom Hall and Vicky Dancer for their secretarial assistance; Christine Smedley, assistant editor at Sage Publications, for her guidance in the editing process; and those publishers who have given permission to use specific copyright material.

These acknowledgments would not be complete without special mention of the fact that the Institute owes its existence, to a considerable degree, to the commitment of two Canadian nurses in particular: Shirley Stinson and Marilynn Wood. It is their courage, support, enthusiasm, trust, and foresight that has largely been responsible for this work coming to fruition in published form.

Prologue: An Invitation to Philosophize

✳

Surely these are exciting times in nursing's history. It appears that we have come to a juncture, a point of realignment, in the development of nursing knowledge. The profession, particularly over the last 2 decades, has become increasingly aware of itself—of its place among the disciplines and of its quest for an organized body of nursing knowledge adequate to the task of guiding its practice and efficiently discharging its obligation to society. The quickening of this self-consciousness came with nursing's disengagement from its handmaiden partnership with medicine. Following that move, nursing felt compelled to eschew all things medical, particularly the disease orientation and the medical model as the source of nursing concepts.

In the 1960s, conceptual frameworks for nursing began to emerge and the thrust toward educational preparation for nurse researchers launched the notion of nursing as a learned profession in the making. In the absence of any sure purpose of its own and the lure of being "scientific," nursing found itself generating scientific knowledge of more and diverse means to an unarticulated end that its practice might serve. One or another end was tentatively adopted; health, well-being, advocacy, caring, coping, self-care, consciousness raising were some among the many proposed.

1

The particularities and generalities of nursing in their most inclusive embodiments, to be had through historical and philosophical inquiry respectively, suffered short shrift. The upshot was that the knowledge being developed was fragmented and ununified. Rumblings from nursing practice were expressions of doubt about the usefulness of the accumulating knowledge. Research-based practice seemed to be more a shibboleth than a clarion call. Crucial philosophic nursing questions began to press in on the profession: Is the research being done by nurse scholars *nursing* research? Is the knowledge being developed *nursing* knowledge? How is the practice of nursing different from that of medicine? Because answers given to philosophic nursing questions affect nursing's artists, researchers, educators, and administrators, all nurses are called upon to philosophize about the nature of nursing, in both its knowledge and practice dimensions. What must the future of nursing be if it continues to focus almost exclusively on nursing science, particularly because only philosophic inquiry is capable of specifying the end to be brought about in nursing practice? Although every nurse interested in or concerned about the future of nursing can and does philosophize about such matters, some must make it their business to become formally prepared to do so, for the well-being of the profession.

This collection of essays constitutes philosophical treatises on the subjects of discourse of the first invitational philosophic nursing conference of the Institute for Philosophical Nursing Research, held in 1989 at the Banff Centre in Alberta, Canada. The reason this particular collection came to be is the same reason that gave birth to the sponsoring Institute: Despite the fact that nursing's progress is as remarkable as it is admirable, nursing is a science in jeopardy and is likely to remain so unless we who serve and shape it take up the challenge posed by identifying and articulating the nature, place, and future of philosophic inquiry in nursing. We must look to philosophical discourse to help us fix the course of nursing's future. It does us little good to agree with Dewey, James, or Adler that philosophy is everybody's business if nursing scholars, present and future, do not make philosophy in nursing their business.

This volume is an attempt to engage the interest, intellect, and will of anyone interested in or concerned about the present and future of nursing as a learned profession, and is particularly aimed at those graduate students who will inherit the cause of nursing as a respectable intellectual discipline and as a practice devoted to efficiently and humanely serving humankind. The essays are offered as an invitation and opportunity to join issue about the need for philosophic inquiry in the nurse's world, in our time and beyond. Each essay is devoted to a topic selected for its relevance as a goad to philosophizing about philosophic inquiry in nursing and as a means of enlarging our understanding of the need for it—the impetus behind both the conference and making the essays widely available. The issue at stake in each topic is one that we believe, left unresolved, harbors an apparent threat to nursing's advancement as a learned profession. It is for that reason that this book sends a message—an invitation—to nurses everywhere, and especially to graduate nursing students, to consider the place and power of philosophic inquiry in disclosing the apparent threat to be just that, apparent; or if real, to dismantle that threat.

It is important that readers recognize that behind each topic addressed is a question to which nurses presently are proposing diverse answers, either in part or in whole. It is for that reason that for two of the topics—the knowledge content of contemporary conceptualizations of nursing and the aim of philosophical inquiry in nursing—two nurse scholars were invited to present their understanding on the matter in question. The reader is at liberty to decide whether more agreement than disagreement obtains between the related essays. The answers articulated in any of the essays are not necessarily the most popular, most sound, or most likely to advance nursing knowledge development. In every instance, however, they do express the different answers offered or positions taken by one or more nursing leaders with respect to the issue under consideration.

We do not believe that nurses anywhere would dispute that diversity, not unity, characterizes nursing thought and knowledge development in contemporary nursing works. Although nurse scholars are prone to speak or write on the same topic, use the same words, or express a common interest in knowledge development, there is very little in their productions to indicate that they share to any great degree a common understanding, a coming-to-terms, that would allow for the minimal topical agreement required before questions can be commonly interpreted, controversies identified, issues debated, and answers commonly agreed upon. Therefore, the conclusions drawn in each treatise of this book are ideas concerning which the reader is called upon to make up her or his own mind—not simply concerning the positions taken by the various authors but, more importantly, about the present condition of nursing knowledge development vis-à-vis those ideas and the need for philosophic inquiry in nursing. With that in mind, the book is divided into three parts: Part One includes essays related to the nature of philosophic inquiry in nursing; Part Two, the place of philosophic inquiry in nursing; and Part Three, the future of philosophic inquiry in nursing. Each part opens with an introduction and guiding questions intended to illuminate the philosophic nursing issue central to that part to help readers think their way through to some resolution of it. The questions are intended to be used for guiding the reader, not as a test of knowledge.

As editors, it is our hope that this collection of essays will succeed in goading readers into philosophizing with colleagues about its important topics, about the positions taken in relation to them by some of the best nursing minds in the field, and about the questions raised. If this happens, then our purpose in putting forward this volume will, in large part, have been met.

PART ONE

The Nature of Philosophic
Inquiry in Nursing

That nursing inquiry has remained essentially scientific in nature until very recently is hardly debatable. Nursing research journals, conferences, projects, and courses have been scientific in orientation. In nursing education, particularly at the master's and doctoral levels, science has reigned supreme. Even now, when nurse educators, researchers, administrators, and clinicians speak of the need for a research-based nursing practice, it is clear that what they have in mind is a practice based on the findings of scientific nursing research. Furthermore, although the nature of scientific nursing research has been the object of inquiry of some nurse scholars, such as Donaldson, Crowley, and Johnson, the nature of scientific research per se has not been a subject of nursing debate. This is no longer the case. Disillusioned with the positivistic approach to science, many nurse researchers, following the social scientists, have turned to other approaches and, in so doing, have stretched the scope of science as traditionally understood.

Previously limited to public, objectively verifiable knowledge, science has been expanded to include, among other things, private knowledge, subjective opinion, and descriptions of lived experience, all of which lie beyond objective verifiability. In attempting to move beyond traditional scientific methods, nurse researchers have not held squarely in view the kind of questions that science is capable of answering and have, at times, unwittingly moved into the realm of questions that only philosophy can answer. In those instances, they have used the scientific mode of inquiry inappropriately, adding to the growing confusion over the nature of philosophic as well as scientific research. It is becoming increasingly clear that the error being made can be traced to a lack of understanding of the nature of the two modes of inquiry, scientific and philosophic.

It is only by attaining understanding of the nature of each mode of inquiry that we can act knowledgeably and thereby downscale the current pervasive misuse of precious time, energy, and other nursing research resources. To this end, Part One is devoted to helping readers philosophize about the nature of philosophic inquiry in nursing. In Chapter 1, the similarities and differences between the scientific and philosophic modes of inquiry are addressed. Chapter 2 focuses more specifically on philosophic nursing inquiry and the kind of nursing questions that can be answered only through philosophic inquiry. Because it is not possible to fully understand the place of philosophic inquiry in nursing (the subject of Part Two) in the absence of knowing whether diversity or unity of thought is to be sought, Part One closes with two essays that address this issue (Chapters 3 and 4). The questions below are designed to help readers make up their own minds on this matter and others regarding the nature of philosophic inquiry in nursing.

Guiding Questions: Making Up Your Own Mind

1. *Are different modes of inquiry necessary in nursing?*

2. *What is the nature, scope, and object of nursing inquiry? Of philosophic nursing inquiry? Of scientific nursing inquiry?*

3. *What are the implications for nursing thought and action of continuing to rely almost entirely on scientific inquiry in nursing?*

4. *What presuppositions underlie and what implications for nursing thought and action flow from the position that philosophic nursing inquiry is nonempirical? Is empirical? That only diversity of thought is to be sought in philosophic nursing inquiry? That only unity of thought is to be sought?*

5. *Can unity and diversity in nursing thought coexist?*

1

Philosophic and Scientific Inquiry: The Interface

✳

HELEN SIMMONS

Let me begin with a question: What is the significance of articulating the interface between philosophic and scientific inquiry for the overriding objective of this conference—namely, to enlarge our understanding of the need for philosophic inquiry in nursing? The answer to that question is this: In effect, if the interface—that is, the common ground constituting thé boundary between these two modes of inquiry—is not made explicit, we will be hard put to appreciate, in each, the *difference that makes a difference.* Since the time of Hume these differences have gone unobserved, giving rise to numerous misconceptions of philosophic inquiry and undermining its importance. In separating the total realm of organized natural knowledge, Hume invoked a principle of division that oversimplified the matter. His distinction between what *is* and what is *not* capable of being tested by appeal to experience set up a disjunction that fixed the order and relation of the disciplines in their modern conception. As a result, abstract reasoning about quantity and number became the sphere of formal or analytic statements, and experimental reasoning about matters of fact or existence became the sphere of empirical or synthetic statements (Jones, 1969, p. 350).

In Hume's conception, as handed down by Emmanuel Kant in his a priori and a posteriori judgments, we meet our epistemologic heritage from the 17th century in all its confusion: Mathematics, science, and history were seen as exhaustively representing all the distinguishable bodies of organized natural knowledge and were nominated the only knowledge worthy of the title. Philosophy was relegated to the plane of second-order questions. Metaphysics, which prior to the 17th century had been accepted as first-order philosophic knowledge, was shunted aside as mere speculation. Philosophers themselves turned their backs on metaphysics, some responding by trying to make philosophy scientific and others by accepting that the only role for philosophy was a therapeutic one, as handmaiden, clarifying or correcting the conceptual errors of other disciplines (Adler, 1965). Under such circumstances, it is not difficult to see why, in contemporary times, when we speak of *knowledge*, if we do not mean *science* we had better explain ourselves; or even worse, why we are prone to seek a scientific or a poetic answer to a philosophic question. This tendency is a clear manifestation of our having attributed sameness where difference in fact prevails. The interface that should obtain has been substituted for by another or, in some instances, has been blurred or displaced entirely.

In this essay, I am contending that if we can get off on the right foot about the interface between these two modes of inquiry, we will not be lured into the knowledge division slough dug by Hume and Kant and therefore should be able to see more clearly in what ways philosophic and scientific inquiry stand to make distinct contributions to the development of an organized body of nursing knowledge. It is my conviction that confusion over the nature and power of these two modes of inquiry is the main source of discord in contemporary thought and in our pursuit of knowledge in contemporary times. Further, I am contending that unless we establish the common ground traversed by these two modes of inquiry, we will not, by any means, be able to appreciate their difference. If we fail in that endeavor, we cannot hope to rid ourselves of the confusion we inherited from the 17th century, which, in my view, has put our epistemological sanity at stake. Examining wherein the two modes of inquiry are the same and, in turn, wherein they are different holds promise, not only of bringing us directly into the polluted waters in which we have been swimming, but also as a springboard for further philosophizing about the need for philosophic inquiry in nursing, the theme of our conference. I now will attempt to disclose the essential nature of the interface between the philosophic and scientific modes of inquiry. I will proceed by adopting, as point of departure, the common conditions both modes must meet in order to be regarded as respectable, intellectual enterprise directed toward and attaining knowledge of reality. I will then discuss their relationship, precisely as modes of inquiry, to each other and to the historical and mathematical modes; describe their tests of truth; and finally, compare their relative usefulness in three dimensions: in their bearing on common-sense opinion, in the sphere of action, and in our coming to understand the world at large.

Throughout this examination, I shall assume a moderate stance arising from common sense. Under it, I shall hold, as assumption, the existence of things apart from the mind and that the mind can know through reflecting on sense data in conformity with reality. We are, after all, seeking knowledge of something outside the mind and not merely of our own ideas. I am proceeding then on the basis that (a) there is knowledge of reality, in the strict sense, requiring for its attainment one or another of the various disciplined modes of inquiry; (b) ordinary knowledge of the sort we gain and use, in everyday experience, also exists; and (c) our experience of the object is neither true nor false—it simply is what it is, and, therefore, experience is not knowledge. In our attempt to better understand the modes of inquiry, it is important that we do not confuse or merge the experiencing of objects with the common-sense propositions we develop concerning them, nor the objects of reality with the ideas by which we grasp them. This is the very point on which 17th century thought got off to a bad start. The upshot of this confusion was to undercut the possibility of knowledge of reality of any sort, philosophic or scientific (Adler, 1974; Regis, 1946, 1959; Simmons & Kikuchi, 1986).

As we know, the condition of all knowledge is abstractness, and the objects of study of the modes of inquiry can be differentiated in terms of their degree of abstractness from matter (Simon, 1943). Philosophical inquiry, being the most abstract, has for its objects the being of everything that is, but only in the light of first causes; whereas, scientific inquiry is obviously less abstract, having for its objects some particular province of being of which it investigates only secondary or proximate principles (Maritain, 1930). Both the material and formal objects of a mode of inquiry serve to distinguish it from another mode of inquiry but, within any given mode, say the scientific mode, only the formal object serves to distinguish one science from another. We can see, for instance, that the health sciences all share the same material object, but what seems not to have been determined is the formal object of each science subsumed. When scientists, using their own mode of inquiry, attempt to answer a philosophic question they have unwittingly confused the material and formal objects of the two modes.[1] That error brings us face to face with the conditions that a mode of inquiry must meet in order to be deemed respectable. Let me proceed then, by setting out some of the more important definitions we will require in order to come to terms about the matter at hand: articulating the interface between the philosophic and scientific modes of inquiry.

A *mode of inquiry* simply put is a formal method required and used by the adherents of a discipline in a deliberate attempt to establish first-order knowledge in the form of testable, verifiable well-founded truths about what is and happens in the world, or about what human beings ought to do and seek. There is, of course, what is called *second-order knowledge:* knowledge *about* the first-order knowledge; however, I intend to limit my remarks primarily to first-order knowledge. I am taking *knowledge* to mean truth about reality as it exists outside the mind and independent of any one mind having knowledge of it. I am defining *science* in terms of its contemporary usage as knowledge of efficient causes, that is, proximate principles of explanation. By *philosophy*, I mean knowledge of first causes or of the highest principles of things in so far as these causes or things belong to the natural, as opposed to the supernatural, order. Whenever I speak of philosophy, I will therefore mean metaphysics, but whatever I say about it can be taken as applicable to the other divisions of philosophy, secundum quid. By *discipline*, I mean an organized body of knowledge in which the propositions are compendious (Adler, 1965; Maritain, 1938).

Mortimer Adler (1965) has set down the common grounds for comparison of the two modes of inquiry as method—but for a different purpose, that of defending philosophy as having a method of its own. Granting that fact, I think it well worth our time to entertain these grounds as first priority in examining the interface, simply because they are the conditions of respectable intellectual enterprise of any sort. In agreement with Aristotle and contemporary moderate realists (Adler, 1965; Maritain, 1930; Wallace, 1983), I accept that mathematics, history, science, and philosophy exhaustively represent all the distinguishable bodies of organized natural knowledge and that each of these fields of inquiry has a method of its own, which aims at and attains knowledge. The modes of inquiry that characterize these disciplines represent all the distinguishable formal modes of inquiry. The existence of common-sense knowledge[2] (and the informal manner through which we go about attaining it) is presupposed.

The conditions that the two modes of inquiry must commonly meet to be held as respectable intellectual enterprise, according to Adler, are six in all. The ones commonly conditioning both the philosophic and scientific modes are these:

1. They must aim at and attain knowledge of reality of the sort we call probable truths.
2. They must in turn have appropriate criteria of truth against which the truth value of their propositions and theories can be legitimately criticized.
3. They must be conducted as public inquiry, meeting all the conditions of public enterprise as such.
4. They must exhibit and exercise relative autonomy in their own domain, being the independent guarantor of the truth of their separate propositions and theories while submitting to their dependency on the rest of human knowledge.
5. They must take responsibility to raise and answer the questions that are strictly their own.

In addition to these five positive conditions, philosophical inquiry alone, because of its special obligation and place in shaping culture and civilization and because of its bearing on common sense, operates under a further negative condition: It must not be esoteric; it must be comprehensible to the average man (pp. 79-80).[3]

I should like here to make three comments on the performance of the practition of these two modes of inquiry. With regard to the first condition, the pursuit of probable (as opposed to certain or absolute) truth, philosophers both among the ancients and moderns have committed some obvious violations of this condition. In contemporary philosophic thought, the almost total abandonment of the pursuit of first-order knowledge and the epistemologizing and psychologizing of knowledge attest to this fact. Science, on the other hand, has its extreme movement away from probable truth in scientists who have taken their theoretical entities to be nothing more than convenient fictions that give us no knowledge of reality whatsoever, probable truths aside. My second comment has to do with moral philosophy in light of the second condition: appropriate criteria of truth. Kant, picking up on Hume's declaration that we could not derive a single practical truth from empirical statements of what is and happens in the world, set the stage for noncognitive ethics and the impossibility of philosophy's attaining probable truths, in its practical aspect of what humans ought to do and seek. Some contemporary thinkers, philosophers and scientists alike, picking up where Kant left off, have denied moral philosophy its proper criterion of truth as established twenty-five hundred years ago by Aristotle (Adler, 1981, pp. 79-81). They have, as consequence, dived headlong into relativism in its subjectivist and idealist form. The consequences for ethics and politics, and in turn for applied and practical science, as we know, stand to deny to practicians in these disciplines sorely needed guidance in the face of the ever increasing power turned loose on the world by modern technology. Obviously, the condition of having an appropriate criterion of truth bears squarely on the use to be made of the products of these two modes of inquiry, as well as on the status of their theoretical concepts as giving or not giving us knowledge of reality or real existents. Both of these points will be revisited later, in the discussion on the usefulness of science and philosophy.

With regard to the fourth and fifth conditions (disciplines exercising relative autonomy and addressing questions of their own), I would only add that it is philosophy that governs, judges, and defends, not only in its own territory of inquiry but in that of science as well (Adler, 1965; Maritain, 1930, pp. 83-92; Wallace, 1983). I will deal with this fact more directly later; for now, suffice it to say that the nature, scope, and object of both disciplines is given in and through philosophic inquiry and that it is these that dictate indirectly and directly the questions properly belonging to each discipline. That much said about the conditions of inquiry as respectable, I leave the reader with this question: How well does contemporary inquiry in nursing measure up against them?

I shall now address the heart of the interface between the philosophic and scientific modes of inquiry. Again, in my estimation it is Adler (1965) who has set out in high relief their sameness and difference. We can do no better, I believe, than to examine his thinking on the matter. In order not to play the philosopher here—to borrow an expression from Jacques Maritain—I shall try to carefully present for you Adler's major conclusions and some of his reasoning on the distinctness of the modes. If I succeed, I believe that what the interface between the philosophic and scientific modes of inquiry essentially is will be adequately disclosed, and any additional considerations will be more easily grasped against that backdrop.

In addressing a comparison of the two modes of inquiry precisely as method, I will begin where Adler, in fact, ends up. He concludes that philosophy contributes in a particular way to first-order knowledge about what is and happens in the world and about what men ought to do and seek. Acceptance of this conclusion, he says, depends principally on two things: (a) acceptance of the existence and distinction between special and common experience, and (b) accepting and "on seeing that common experience can serve the philosopher in ways that are strictly comparable to the ways in which special experience serves the scientist" (p. 119). It follows that accepting his conclusions further presupposes the distinction, expressed earlier, between knowledge and experience and, additionally, between experience and inquiry.

By special experience, Adler means the experience we attain by deliberately investigating, contriving a situation in which to observe and collect data. By common experience, he means the core of those experiences all humans have without a single effort at investigating anything, and he does not mean those experiences that are different for this or that person because they are dependent on individual differences in constitution or attainments or circumstances of time and place. For Adler, "experience does not consist of assertions; it is neither true nor false; it is simply whatever it is. In contrast, knowledge (doxa) consists of assertions which may be either true or false" (p. 102) and is based on experience. Inquiry itself is either empirical (based in experience) or not. Adler defines *investigation* as "the process of deliberately making observations either for the express purpose of answering certain questions or solving certain problems or for the purpose of testing hypotheses, theories, conclusions or conjectures" (p. 101). Accordingly, a mode of inquiry is investigative, if it proceeds by deliberately making observations for one or more of these purposes.

In setting out the sameness and difference among the modes of inquiry, Adler uses three principles of division: (a) investigative versus noninvestigative in method; (b) testability versus nontestability of their products by appeal to experience; and (c) their objects as particular versus general, that is, as "singularly determined in space and time versus objects not so determined" (pp. 114-117).

Between philosophic and scientific inquiry the common ground is their dependence on experience for developing their concepts, forming their questions, and testing their propositions and theories. Also, their objects of inquiry are general, not particular; therefore, their questions about what is and happens in the world are about universals. Both develop propositions or conclusions that belong in the sphere of synthetic statements (i.e., statements that are falsifiable by appeal to experience); in short, both modes are empirical. Both bear a relationship to investigation per se—in the case of science a positive relationship and in philosophy a negative one. (To not be investigative, let me hasten to remark, is no sin. It does not diminish the possibility of attaining truth by the philosophic mode of inquiry.) This, then, sets us out on the path of their difference: Science is investigative, and philosophy is not; science depends on special experience, philosophy on common experience—for engendering their concepts and for the falsifiability of their propositions and theories. Another difference is that philosophic inquiry, unlike scientific, can and does answer second-order questions about the semantics, syntax, and logic involved in first-order knowledge about universals, about the questions and answers that both science and philosophy pose. The conclusions that second-order philosophy arrives at belong in the sphere of analytic statements and cannot be tested by appeal to experience of any sort, special or common. Both second-order and first-order philosophy use armchair thinking because of their dependence on common experience; as method, philosophy alone requires no special investigation or experiments—no arrays of data—merely the common experience open to anyone and everyone (pp. 111-119).

In summary, in their convergence, both modes of inquiry are dependent on experience for their concepts, postulates, and the falsifiability of their products in the sphere of synthetic (empirical) statements; both have general objects; and both, therefore, raise questions about universals. The two modes diverge completely in the fact that science is investigative and dependent on special experience. Philosophy is discursive, noninvestigative, depends on common experience, and (with regard to its second-order products in the sphere of analytic [formal] statements) is not falsifiable by appeal to any sort of experience, special or common. The essence of the scientific mode is its nature as investigative; the essence of the philosophic mode is its dependence on common experience.

In contrast, the historical mode is set apart from both the philosophic and the scientific mode, in light of the fact that its objects of inquiry are particular and past events and its questions are about singulars. It is similar to scientific inquiry in being investigative, but the conclusions of science are general statements about classes of objects as opposed to those of history, which are about singular happenings or existences that are not present and not capable of direct observation, but only indirectly so (Adler, 1965, p. 106). It is similar to both philosophic and scientific inquiry in being empirical. Mathematics, on the other hand, is separated from both science and first-order philosophy by the fact that its products fall in the sphere of analytical (formal) statements that are *not* falsifiable by appeal to any experience and does not have objects of inquiry that are mutable, sensible, physical, or matter of fact (pp. 108-111). The alignment of mathematics with second-order philosophy is complete on all counts. Because of philosophy's dependence on common experience and science's on special investigation, it follows that the man in the street is more or less competent to make up his own mind about matters philosophic but not so about scientific ones. This fact, I believe, has a direct bearing on the responsibility question addressed by Dr. Schlotfeldt in Chapter 9.

Let us now proceed to another aspect of the interface: the tests of truth appropriate to both science and philosophy. They are called the *empirical* and *logical* tests. The empirical test subjects the products of inquiry to falsifiability in experience, special *and* common,[4] and in it only the negative result is decisive. The logical test is applied to theories not so falsified, to determine their comparative internal consistency, comprehensiveness, and elegance within the given field of inquiry (Adler, 1965, pp. 154-157).

In addition to the empirical and logical tests of truth, common to both modes of inquiry, philosophic inquiry addressed in its practical branch allows for what Adler calls the *is-ought test*, in which philosophic knowledge of what is or happens in the world and philosophic knowledge of what ought to be done or sought serve as a test of each other's soundness in judging the relative truth of competing philosophic theories. And, when they conflict, sound *ought-knowledge* (because of the primacy given it by common sense) is arbitrator over sound *is-knowledge* (p. 196). Finally, philosophic inquiry applies one further test to its products or theories when relevant scientific knowledge (or knowledge from any other discipline) must be taken into account: the *mixed-question test* (p. 149). Given scientific knowledge that appears to conflict with common-sense opinion, philosophic analysis either demonstrates the conflict to be apparent only or is called upon to resolve the conflict if it is genuine.

So much for the tests of truth common to both modes of inquiry and those unique to the philosophic mode—they will surface again in the discussion on the usefulness of the two modes. Here, the question I leave the reader with is this: What is the relevance of these tests for examining the propositions asserted to be true in contemporary conceptualizations of nursing? Now, as a final consideration of the interface, I will put forward the usefulness of the two modes of inquiry in three dimensions: in their bearing on common-sense opinion; in the world of action (i.e., in seeking, making, and doing); and in our general understanding of the world.

In their bearing on common-sense opinion, the roles of the two modes of inquiry are almost totally distinct (Adler, 1965; Maritain, 1938). Scientific inquiry corrects and extends common-sense opinion. In its correcting function, it operates where error is due to the inadequacy of the common experience on which the common-sense opinion rests, and investigation is needed because the detail required to correct the opinion is beyond the reach of common experience (e.g., in matters concerning the shape of the earth, sensory illusion, the comparative strength of metals, and so on). When scientific inquiry extends common-sense opinion, it does so where common-sense opinion is correct, as far as it goes, but does not go far enough. Obvious examples of such extension are the manner in which and in what amounts ordinary substances, such as sugar and salt, have a deleterious effect on our body's organs; or what all is involved in forecasting the weather; or in answering questions about matters that do not even occur to common sense. All this said, it is important to remember that following investigation, our experience of such matters remains as it was prior to investigation.

Philosophic inquiry, on the other hand, corrects and defends common-sense opinion. It corrects common-sense opinion where common experience is adequate and where investigation is impossible. It does so, for example, in such matters as good and evil, right and wrong, duties and obligations, virtues and vices, life's purpose or goal, rights and justice, the good society, the just economy or polity, war and peace, and so on. Wherever philosophy acts to correct or defend common-sense opinion, it is a matter of the inadequacy of understanding the common experience underlying the opinion. Where philosophical inquiry sets a defense of common-sense opinion, it is usually in instances where some theory reduces such opinion to linguistic habit, or dismisses it entirely as illusory or as tautological, as is wont to be the case in the claim of circularity levelled at the self-evident truths learned by sensitive intuition by the adherents of nominalistic, materialistic, atomistic, or empiricist approaches to knowledge attainment (Adler, 1965, pp. 134-146; Adler, 1971; Maritain, 1930, chap. 8; Maritain, 1938).

Let me now examine the usefulness of these two modes of inquiry in the sphere of action. It is appropriate, because of the distinct contributions of each, to speak to the major divisions of the two fields of inquiry or disciplines they serve. Each has three major divisions. Science is divided into pure science (natural and social), practical science, and applied science. Pure science is purely speculative scientific knowledge about what is and happens in the world. Practical science is science only in an improper sense in that it is practical or productive know-how knowledge, a special type of knowledge required to put is-knowledge to use. Practical know-how is knowledge involved in putting is-knowledge to use in the sphere of human conduct, both individual and social. Productive know-how is the knowledge required to put is-knowledge to use in making things or achieving various effects. Know-how is predominantly art—the rules of the art of making or doing written declaratively: what the Greeks called *techne*. Pure science is turned into applied science by the addition of productive know-how and is manifest in technology and other applications (Adler, 1965, p. 183).

Philosophy, on the other hand, has as its major divisions speculative philosophy, normative philosophy, and logic. Speculative philosophy is usually subdivided into metaphysics, natural philosophy, and criticism (or epistemology) and is philosophic knowledge about what is or happens in the world. Normative philosophy is knowledge about what "ought to be" sought or done and made and has the three subdivisions of ethics, economics, and politics. Logic, the third major division of philosophy, has a very special role in that it is necessary as preparatory to proceeding effectively in any discipline (Wallace, 1977).

We are now in a position to examine the usefulness of philosophic and scientific inquiry in the world of both action and production. It seems reasonable to conclude that in that world the measure of their usefulness is that of their respective products—in short, the usefulness of science and of philosophy. It should be pointed out that in modern times, *action* has been used to cover both doing and making; thereby unwittingly introducing error into our thinking. It is both possible and profitable to keep these notions separate in the way that Adler, following Aristotle, does. Here, I will use action to mean only "doing"—that is, what we do in the conduct of our individual lives and social affairs—and *production* for conduct in making things.

When it comes to determining efficient means and what practicable means are available to do and make things, science has it over philosophy hands down. For those purposes, philosophy is totally useless in both its speculative and practical divisions. I am not sure who said it first, but, put succinctly, "philosophy builds no bridges and bakes no cakes." Science, on the other hand, gives us better and better means—more and more power to control, manipulate, and predict. Scientific knowledge of what is and what happens in the world is indirectly put to work; that is, its use is mediated by productive and practical know-how. The rules of art, both productive and practical (for making and doing) are etched out by science. In doing and making, we need both moral ought (and ought-not) knowledge plus practical and productive know-how. Normative philosophic inquiry supplies the one and scientific inquiry supplies the other (Adler, 1965, p. 188). With regard to telling us what we ought to seek, whether we ought to pursue this or that goal, use this or that available efficient means, science is as useless in these respects as philosophy is for building bridges and baking cakes. Or, to raise it to the level of hotter contemporary conflicts on issues—such as in what natural processes we should use our scientific technology to intervene, to modify or to subdue; what military pursuits we ought to undertake; whether we should or should not enter space to travel or pollute—on all this, scientific inquiry can do nothing other than remain silent. Only normative philosophic inquiry can help us here, and only if it applies an appropriate means of establishing and testing practical truths. With regard to the latter point, noncognitive ethics and Kant's golden-rule imperative, lacking such means, will not carry us safely across the street.

In summary then, in the practical-productive order, the products of scientific inquiry give us more and more productive power, and philosophic inquiry is called upon to give us better and better direction, or at least good direction in the conduct of our individual and social affairs. Perhaps, here, it is important to recall that action and production happen in the particular concrete situation and, because the objects of inquiry are general in both modes of inquiry, it requires moral virtue and prudence to complete our scientific and philosophic knowledge for use in the particular case. The question for nursing inquiry that I will leave the reader with here is this: If nursing science is practical science, as I believe it is, what is the scope of its dependence on normative philosophic inquiry, and how direct or indirect is that dependence?

I will now proceed to examine the usefulness of science and philosophy in helping us to understand the world. Their difference in usefulness as products "corresponds to their methods as modes of inquiry" (Adler, 1965, p. 188) and so, indirectly, is a reflection of the usefulness of the modes themselves—their usefulness in the manner in which each renders the nature of things intelligible, in the form of first-order knowledge of what is and happens in the world. In the light of the philosophy of science and, therefore, in intimacy with the mixed-question test of truth, we are faced with the conditions of possible or even likely conflict between scientific and philosophic theory. The reason is that philosophers and scientists, as enquirers into what is and happens in the world, frequently take different positions on the nature and existence of reality and on whether or not we can attain knowledge of it, in the form of probable truths. Regarding mixed questions, when both scientific and philosophic theories purport to extend or elucidate common-sense opinion, then the conflict could be real. In that case, answers to mixed questions require that we avoid contradiction in the theory or conclusions, because both modes of inquiry are aiming at knowledge that arrives at probable truths or relatively true descriptions of reality. We are obligated, therefore, to relate what is asserted in the results of the two modes of inquiry

(p. 216). Recall that science answers the questions that cannot be answered without investigation, philosophy answers those that cannot be answered by investigation, and the mixed-question test applies only to the truths attained by the philosophic mode. On that account, one measure of the soundness and, therefore, the usefulness of the products or theory developed through the philosophic mode, is the theory's "ability to reconcile what truth there is in scientific theory with what truth there is in common-sense opinion and in the philosophic elucidation of that opinion" (Adler, 1965, p. 224) under conditions of apparent conflict between those truths. For example, if common-sense opinion defended by philosophic inquiry is demonstrated not to be illusory, we would be forced on empirical grounds to reject the philosophic doctrine of atomistic materialism of common-existent physicals in everyday life (chairs, tables, bottles of wine) as nothing but matter in motion and to reject instrumentalism, which holds such things to be "convenient fictions." Or, to take another example, the empiricist view (or *sense-data theory*) as a theory of experience can be demonstrated, through philosophic defense of common sense, to be wholly unacceptable—inadequate to explain our everyday experience. It should not escape us here that philosophies of science are philosophic theories; they are not scientific theories (p. 225).

The *relative* soundness of one philosophic theory as opposed to another, then, depends on which presents a more satisfactory resolution of conflicts arising in mixed questions. I do not mean to say here that science cannot contribute at all to that resolution. Rather, the contribution has to be indirect or mediated by the usefulness of products of scientific inquiry to philosophy. Maritain (1930) states that there are four uses a philosopher should make of science:

(i) to illustrate aptly his principles, (ii) to confirm his conclusions, (iii) to interpret, throw light upon, and assimilate, the assured results of the sciences so far as questions of philosophy are involved. And finally he should use the affirmations of science (iv) to refute objections and errors which claim support from its results. (p. 91)

This requires that any of us intending to become philosophic inquirers should first undergo training in scientific inquiry in order to be able to spot pseudoscientific conclusions. Otherwise, one might not, for instance, recognize and debunk, as pseudoscientific, (erroneous) theories put forward by any number of social scientists to supplant conclusions that can only be drawn through philosophic inquiry.

In concluding which mode of inquiry gives us a better understanding of what is and happens in the world—the philosophic or scientific mode—we are compelled, I believe, to agree with Adler (1965). We must choose the former because (a) only philosophic inquiry can resolve conflicts between its discipline and other disciplines; (b) the different views of science are philosophic views so that understanding science itself requires philosophic inquiry; (c) only philosophic inquiry can give us an overall understanding from elementary common experience to ultimate causes in things; (d) philosophical inquiry gives us understanding of the world as known through science and, more immediately, through commonsense knowledge; and (e) over and above these theoretical insights into the world at large, through inquiry in practical matters, it directs us in the conduct of our individual and social affairs, in the maintenance of the species and the advancement, as opposed to the destruction, of civilization (pp. 225-227). The attitude of scientific inquiry in deciding these practical matters is "indifference."

In closing, I will pose one final question regarding nursing inquiry: What is the rightful place of philosophic nursing inquiry in helping us understand what is and what happens in the world of nursing and what nurses, as such, ought to do and seek?

In this essay, relying in large part on the work of Mortimer Adler and of other moderate realists, I have attempted to make explicit the major features that characterize the common boundary between philosophic and scientific inquiry: the characteristics conditioning them as respectable intellectual enterprise directed toward and attaining knowledge of reality; their relationship precisely as modes of inquiry; their tests of truth; and their relative usefulness, direct and indirect, as seen through the usefulness of the knowledge each attains. As to whether or not the common ground has been adequately charted, or whether or not apprehending what the interface consists of can help us more clearly see the distinct contributions each mode of inquiry can make to the development of an organized body of nursing knowledge, each reader is, of course, charged with making up his/her own mind.

NOTES

1. "The formal object is the aspect under which it [inquiry] apprehends its material object and that which it studies primarily and 'intrinsically' and in reference to which it studies everything else; that, for philosophy, is the first cause in things. The material object is simply the subject-matter; that, for philosophy, is everything that exists" (Maritain, 1930, p. 79). The formal object as that "in reference to which" everything else is studied is, I believe, what nurses mean when they speak of "the nursing perspective." In saying this, I am disagreeing with Adam (see Chapter 5).

2. By *common-sense knowledge* of the world, I (following Adler, 1965) mean the aggregate of common-sense opinions or beliefs that are *not* obtained in a methodical, self-critical manner, but nonetheless have more definite justification than mere opinion. Common sense itself is simply our tendency to form opinions on the basis of common experiences and without any intention to pursue knowledge—common experience being that which we undergo simply by being alive, the core of which is the same for all humans across time and place. Common human experience (such as waking, sleeping, laughing, crying, breathing, touching, etc.), then, yields common-sense opinions that taken in aggregate constitute what we call common-sense knowledge (Adler, 1965, pp. 131-146, especially footnotes 1, 3, and 4).

3. Existentialists, phenomenologists, instrumentalists, analysts, and British empiricists all would be forced to reject one or more of these conditions on the basis of the presuppositions they espouse regarding nature itself or the nature of man, or of knowledge and truth (Adler, 1965, pp. 50-71).

4. The failure of Popper (1965) and others to distinguish between common and special experience erroneously limits the method and products of philosophic inquiry to the level of second-order therapeutic enterprise (Adler, 1965; Coffey, 1917; Maritain, 1938).

REFERENCES

Adler, M. J. (1965). *The conditions of philosophy.* New York: Atheneum.

Adler, M. J. (1971). *The common sense of politics.* New York: Holt, Rinehart & Winston.

Adler, M. J. (1974). Little errors in the beginning. *The Thomist, 38,* 27-48.

Adler, M. J. (1981). *Six great ideas.* New York: Macmillan.

Coffey, P. (1917). *Epistemology* (Vol. 2). London: Longmans, Green.

Jones, W. T. (1969). *A history of western philosophy: Hobbes to Hume* (2nd ed.). New York: Harcourt Brace Jovanovich.

Maritain, J. (1930). *An introduction to philosophy* (1979 ed.). New York: Sheed & Ward.

Maritain, J. (1938). *Degrees of knowledge* (B. Wall, Trans.). Glasgow: The University Press.

Popper, K. (1965). *The logic of scientific discovery.* New York: Harper & Row.

Regis, L. (1946). *St. Thomas and epistemology.* Milwaukee: Marquette University Press.

Regis, L. (1959). *Epistemology.* New York: Macmillan.

Simmons, H., & Kikuchi, J. (1986). New frontiers in nursing research: Errors at the cutting edge [Abstract]. In S. M. Stinson, J. C. Kerr, P. Giovannetti, P. Field,

& J. MacPhail (Eds.), *New frontiers in nursing research. Proceedings of the International Nursing Research Conference* (p. 337). Edmonton, Alberta, Canada: University of Alberta.

Simon, Y. R. (1943). Maritain's philosophy of the sciences. *The Thomist, 5,* 85-102.

Wallace, W. A. (1977). *The elements of philosophy.* New York: Alba House.

Wallace, W. A. (1983). *From a realist point of view: Essays on the philosophy of science.* Lanham, MD: University Press of America.

2

Nursing Questions That Science Cannot Answer

✳

JUNE F. KIKUCHI

Science—what nursing questions can it answer? What nursing questions can it *not* answer? Indeed, are there *any* nursing questions that science, as a mode of inquiry, cannot answer? Certainly, given the tremendous success of science to date and the omnipresence of science, it is easy to be lured into thinking that we not only can, but must, turn to science for answers to all of our questions. That we have been so lured is clear: Science reigns supreme in the world of nursing research.

That science dominates nursing research is not problematic—in fact, because nursing as a discipline is a science, it is to be expected. What *is* of concern is that nurses are erroneously subjecting to scientific study nursing questions that are nonscientific—beyond the scope of science to answer. This misuse of science is clearly evident in the scientific studies being conducted using the grounded theory method (à la Glaser and Strauss) to answer philosophical nursing questions such as "What is the nature of nursing?" and "What is the nature of the nurse-client relationship?" Adequate answers to such questions will not be forthcoming until they are recognized as philosophical in nature and are pursued philosophically, not scientifically.

It is my contention that the present misuse of science by nurses, and its attendant consequences, will persist unless and until philosophy, as a mode of inquiry, is allowed to take its rightful place in the nurse's world, for it is only by philosophizing that we can ascertain the kind of nursing question that is (and those that are not) amenable to scientific study. In this essay, with the hope of goading us into philosophizing about those nursing questions that science cannot answer, I present a position that is grounded in the *moderate realist* view of reality—a view that in my estimation is the most tenable and that nurses must adopt if nursing is to have a future as a learned profession (i.e., as a societal institution with an organized body of knowledge and with activities of its own, which exists to serve a practical end, a "particular human good" (Maritain, 1930, p. 111). I say this because in this view the existence of reality independent of the mind is supposed: objective reality with natural forms, boundaries, and orders, against which the truth of propositions can be tested, making possible the attainment of knowledge (in the form of probable truth) of reality. The importance of this supposition becomes evident as this essay unfolds.

In putting forward my position, given the time constraint and the theme of the conference, I have decided to focus on only one kind of nursing question that science cannot answer: the philosophical. Let me begin by defining three key terms: nursing question, science, and philosophy. Other key terms will be defined as they arise.

What is a nursing question? An answer to this philosophical nursing question presupposes an answer to another philosophical nursing question: What is the nature of nursing? As we all know, in searching for an adequate definition of nursing, we have hit dangerous potholes and landmines. Given that we are without adequate answers to both of these questions and that in this essay I do not intend to seek such answers, in order that I might proceed, permit the term *nursing question* to be incompletely defined as follows: questions that are controlled by the end or goal of nursing practice. To define it in terms of the end or goal of nursing practice seems proper because, as Wallace (1977) correctly states, "That which is final in the place of action is the cause of all the activity leading to it" (p. 157). I acknowledge that for many purposes this definition would not be useful, in that it includes the undefined term *nursing*; however, it is adequate to the task at hand.

Because of the various ways in which the terms *science* and *philosophy* are used, it is problematic, especially in epistemological treatises, if these terms are left undefined. Unless otherwise specified, in speaking of science and philosophy, I am referring to specific modes of inquiry, the aim of which is to attain knowledge, in the form of probable truth, about reality—a world of real existences that exists outside and independent of our minds (Adler, 1965). As a mode of inquiry, science inquires into the phenomenal aspects of reality, philosophy into those aspects that transcend the phenomenal (Maritain, 1930). An elaboration of this distinction follows in the next section.

In agreement with Adler (1965), I am taking probable truths to be truths that are "(1) testable by reference to evidence, (2) subject to rational criticism, and either (3) corrigible and rectifiable or (4) falsifiable" (p. 28). Such truths are distinctively different from necessary truths, which are characterized by certainty and finality, such as self-evident truths; and from statements we make from time to time about our own subjective experiences, such as "I feel ill," which unless we are prevaricating also have certitude and finality for us when we make them (p. 26). Furthermore, probable truths are not to be confused with mere opinion, which is "irresponsible, unreliable, unfounded, unreasonable" (p. 29).

Having defined some key terms, let me now present my position. I will proceed by first establishing the essential distinction between scientific and philosophical questions. Then I will consider the kinds of questions that constitute the realm of philosophical nursing questions—a realm beyond science's investigative power.

SCIENTIFIC AND PHILOSOPHICAL QUESTIONS

Why is it that science cannot answer philosophical questions? Is it merely that science does not yet have the means to do so? What if we devised additional scientific methods? It is my contention that no scientific method would help us here. Philosophical questions are questions regarding aspects of reality that are not amenable to scientific study in that they transcend the material. Being metaphysical, they lie outside science's realm—the realm of the phenomenal (Maritain, 1930). Scientific questions, then, are questions regarding the phenomenal (material) aspects of reality. Let me try to make this distinction between philosophical and scientific questions clear, by calling upon the work of Aristotle (as interpreted by Wallace, 1977) concerning the matter of change.

In grappling with the perplexing philosophical problem of change (how it is that things change and yet remain the same), Aristotle reasoned that two coexisting intrinsic principles were operative in every change: (a) *form*, the principle that actuates matter (i.e., that makes a thing be what it is); and (b) *matter*, the principle that receives the actuation (i.e., that of which a thing is made). Now, there are (a) two kinds of form: substantial and accidental, and (b) two kinds of matter: primary and secondary. *Substantial form* actuates *primary matter* (or what may be thought of as undifferentiated protomatter) making it *be* a thing of a specific kind or essence (such as "a dog" or "a human"), or what is called *secondary matter*. Operating on this secondary matter (i.e., the actuated primary matter), *accidental forms* qualify it to be this way or that in certain respects (such as its color and size), resulting in, for example, "a large, brown dog."

According to Aristotle, *substantial change* entails a change of substantial form; in such a change, a thing wholly becomes a thing of another kind, such as takes place at death. *Accidental change* entails a change of accidental form(s); in this kind of change, a thing changes in one or more respects while retaining its substantial form, such as takes place when a baby grows. To illustrate, as a baby grows, it changes only in an accidental way. For example, it becomes larger in size, and its hair color and tone of voice may change; however, throughout such changes, the baby does not change substantially—it retains the human form or essence that it had at conception (albeit in potency) and will retain until death.

Now—relating Aristotle's work to the matter at hand—science concerns itself with the accidental or phenomenal; philosophy with the substantial or nonphenomenal. Science has the power to answer questions regarding the accidental aspects of things (e.g., questions about how babies change as they grow); however, it has no power to answer questions regarding the substantial aspect of things (the essence of things, such as the babies' humanness). Questions about essences or forms per se, the metaphysical aspects of things, lie in the metaphysical realm, a realm addressed by philosophy.

When we are faced with philosophical questions (speculative questions regarding metaphysical aspects of reality and the normative questions grounded in them), science's investigative observational and measurement tools are useless. We have no recourse but to use that wonderful power that we possess—reason—which, unfortunately, seems to be taking a backseat to feelings lately. Moderate realism, a common-sense philosophy, holds that by reflecting on and discursively analyzing our common-sense knowledge (that which we know, not through investigation, but by common sense in light of common experience available to all of us by virtue of being awake), answers to philosophical questions can be attained that are empirically grounded and, furthermore, do not conflict with our common-sense knowledge (Adler, 1965). If you will recall, I have grounded my position on the matter of nursing questions that science cannot answer in moderate realist thought. Therefore, all of its tenets are presupposed, the most important being that philosophy can attain probable truths about reality through the use of reason.

Having made the essential distinction between philosophical and scientific questions, let us turn to the nurse's world and consider the structure of the realm of philosophical nursing questions: philosophical questions controlled by the end or goal of nursing practice.

PHILOSOPHICAL NURSING QUESTIONS

An examination of the contemporary nursing literature (apart from an examination of the reported methods used by nurse researchers) might lead one to conclude that philosophical nursing questions are of two kinds: ethical and epistemological. Would we be correct in so concluding? To answer this question, it may be fruitful to look first at ethical nursing questions: There seems to be little dispute within nursing that these questions are philosophical in nature.

Ethical Nursing Questions

In the last decade, numerous publications have appeared in which the term *nursing ethics* has been used, leading one to conclude that the realm of philosophical nursing questions includes, at minimum, ethical nursing questions. In point of fact, ethical nursing knowledge is the only kind of philosophical nursing knowledge identified by Carper (1975), Jacobs-Kramer and Chinn (1988), Schlotfeldt (1988), and Walker (1971) in their conceptualizations of nursing knowledge. Furthermore, it is equated by the latter two authors with "nursing philosophy" and "philosophy of nursing," respectively. However, as a recent issue of *Advances in Nursing Science* devoted to ethical issues (Chinn, 1989) indicates, a point yet to be resolved is whether or not there are, indeed, ethical nursing questions—whether or not the ethical principles that guide nursing activities are attained by nursing ethics or by ethics proper.

It would seem that because ethics proper addresses questions about what is good to do and to seek, specifically as human, in order to attain a good human life, nursing ethics would be required to address questions about what is good to do and to seek, specifically as nurses, in order to attain the end or goal of nursing practice—in short, to answer ethical nursing questions. It would also seem that given the nature of ethics proper and of nursing ethics, the latter derives ethical nursing principles from principles that the former has worked out. If so, nursing ethics, as knowledge, would not (as the previously mentioned nurse scholars claim) consist of ethical theories or professional codes of behavior: the former would be presupposed and the latter derived from nursing ethics (ethical nursing principles).

Let me hasten to add that nursing politics would also be required to address questions about what nursing, as a political institution, ought to do and to seek in order to meet its social mission—to answer political nursing questions. As is the case for nursing ethics, answers to political nursing questions, it would seem, are derived from principles that politics proper (i.e., political philosophy) has worked out.

Moving along to epistemological questions, let us consider the existence of epistemological nursing questions.

Epistemological Nursing Questions

As is the case for nursing ethics, it would seem that because epistemology proper addresses questions regarding human knowledge in general (its nature, scope, and object), nursing epistemology would be required to address questions regarding nursing knowledge (its nature, scope, and object)—epistemological nursing questions. That these questions do exist and have been addressed by nurse scholars with increasing frequency is evident, for example, in the compilation of papers published in *Perspectives on Nursing Theory* by Nicoll (1986).

Again, it would seem that, as is the case for nursing ethics and nursing politics, answers to epistemological nursing questions are derived from principles that epistemology proper has worked out. It is important to note that this would only be the case if epistemology were conceived as giving us new knowledge. It would not be the case if the position taken up by some contemporary philosophers, such as Adler (1965), were adopted: the position that epistemology "gives us no new knowledge, it serves only to clarify what we already know . . . [it gives us] only a better understanding of the facts already known by other disciplines" (Adler, 1965, p. 47).[1]

In adhering to the positive position—that epistemology proper and nursing epistemology give us new knowledge—it then becomes possible to raise epistemological nursing questions with a future, the asking and answering of which will bring us ever closer to identifying and developing the body of nursing knowledge required for attaining the end of nursing practice. What are these questions? Because the focus of the conference is epistemological in nature, it may be helpful to identify some of these questions and also concerns related to them.

Some critical questions come immediately to mind: Is there such an entity as nursing knowledge? If so, what is its nature? What are its parameters? What is its object? There are those who have dismissed these questions, saying that it is pointless to ask them because there are no genuine boundaries to knowledge of any sort. Others who have tried to answer them, but without success, have dismissed them, saying that it is a waste of time and energy to continue to struggle with them because the answers are too elusive. Still others, myself included, contend that these questions are not so easily dismissed. They continually crop up in our interactions with other disciplines, funding agencies, the public, the media, health care institutions, and so forth. I submit that we must *not* try to escape asking and answering these questions but rather face them squarely. Only by so doing can we attain the knowledge that will ensure that the research endeavors of nurses directly and essentially serve the end or goal of nursing.

In addressing the aforementioned epistemological nursing questions, three epistemological distinctions must be made. It is of concern that these distinctions are not being made in the nursing literature. If made, the confusion that currently pervades our thinking stands to be replaced by clarity.

First, a distinction must be made between (a) the knowledge nurses use in order to nurse, and (b) the knowledge that comprises the body of nursing knowledge. Are these synonymous? Some nurses certainly seem to be treating them as such. I contend that they are not synonymous and that the latter is part of the former— the knowledge that comprises the body of nursing knowledge is only one kind of knowledge that nurses use in order to nurse. Furthermore, it is only the body of nursing knowledge that nursing is responsible for developing. Nursing is not responsible for developing the other kinds of knowledge nurses use, such as the preclinical and personal knowledge nurses use to do their work. By *preclinical knowledge* I mean that knowledge that nurses use or take on as assumption, which lies outside their discipline; by *personal knowledge* I mean that knowledge described by Carper (1975) as subjective, incommunicable, publicly unverifiable, and therefore not possessed by anyone other than the one whose direct knowledge it is. Indeed, how could nursing be held responsible for developing such private knowledge?

Another distinction requiring our attention is the difference between (a) private ways of knowing, such as intuiting, that may contribute to the development of nursing's body of knowledge but *only* indirectly; and (b) public ways of knowing, such as scientizing and philosophizing, that stand to contribute directly. Private ways of knowing serve only as possible means to public ways of knowing—ways that possess the power to make available, for public examination and testing, their methods and resultant evidence and, thereby, directly serve the development of knowledge. How can intuition be other than an indirect contributor, given that it is a private experience?

The failure to make these two distinctions may be a result, in part, of the failure to make a third distinction: the difference between (a) that which is private, and (b) that which is public. According to Adler (1985), that which is private "belongs to one individual alone and cannot possibly be shared directly by anyone else" (p. 10); and that which is public is "common to two or more individuals" (p. 10). Private ways of knowing and knowledge, then, are subjective: "differ[ent] from one person to another and . . . exclusively the possession of one individual and no one else" (p. 9). They are incommunicable and publicly unverifiable. Public ways of knowing and knowledge, on the other hand, are objective: "the same for me, for you, and for anyone else" (p. 9). They are communicable and publicly verifiable. Of late, nurses (e.g., Carper, 1975; Jacobs-Kramer & Chinn, 1988; Kidd & Morrison, 1988; Schultz & Meleis, 1988) seem not to be paying heed to these three distinctions in setting down their conceptualizations of nursing knowledge. Consequently, when a reference is made to nursing knowledge, at times it is impossible to determine if the referent is (a) the knowledge that nurses possess and/or use, or (b) the knowledge that lies within the body of nursing knowledge. Perhaps the failure to make these distinctions is intentional in that it is being presupposed that there are no differences in kind (i.e., no natural forms and boundaries) in reality, only differences in degree. Such a presupposition would explain nurses' growing reluctance to differentiate between (a) nursing's body of knowledge, and (b) those of other disciplines; and between (a) ways of knowing and knowledge that are public and objective, and (b) those that are private and subjective. It seems likely that this presupposition may be operative, because questions about whether or not nursing knowledge is borrowed or unique seem to have disappeared from the nursing literature and to have been replaced with questions about the knowledge that nurses possess and use.

Let me move on now to another kind of philosophical nursing question, a kind that is, unfortunately, neglected in the nursing epistemological literature: the ontological.

Ontological Nursing Questions

It is problematic that in contemporary conceptualizations of nursing knowledge, for the most part, no reference is made to ontological nursing knowledge: knowledge about nursing as a *being*. Are we to take, from this absence, that it is being presupposed, as identified earlier, that there are no differences of kind in reality, only differences of degree? I suspect this may be so because, if such were the case, no ontological nursing questions regarding the nature, scope, and object of nursing would be asked. However, we do ask such questions. How would those who deny the existence of ontological and ontological nursing questions account for the occurrence of such questions? I suspect that they would identify them as scientific, in which case they would also claim that answers to such questions would be found in the science of nursing, both of which are errors.

I submit that if ontological nursing questions are treated as scientific and "answered" scientifically, then we will attain merely knowledge of nursing as it exists phenomenally or accidentally and as it appears to us. But then, if it is being presupposed that there are no natural forms and boundaries in reality, this is the end of the line. To acknowledge the existence of ontological nursing questions and the possibility of attaining philosophical knowledge of nursing as it exists substantially, as a being, would require our holding the presupposition that natural forms and boundaries, differences of kind, do exist in reality. In my estimation, to do otherwise is suicidal. If only differences of degree exist, then we are left with no universal natural truths or order and with having to impose meaning and order on the world. This bodes ill in terms of knowledge development, because all we can possibly attain in that case is a plurality of mere opinions, which may be upheld by consensus or by what can be referred to as "might makes right."

As is the case for nursing ethics, nursing politics, and nursing epistemology, it would seem that answers to ontological nursing questions are derived from principles that ontology proper has worked out. It would also seem that because ontology proper addresses questions about being *qua* being, nursing ontology would be required to address questions about nursing as a being—in short, to answer ontological nursing questions, questions about the substantial nature, scope, and object of nursing. It is imperative that we identify these aspects of nursing, because without doing so it is impossible to identify the substantial nature, scope, and object of nursing knowledge. Furthermore, it would be impossible to establish the end of nursing practice, because the object in nursing thought is the end in nursing action. Without knowledge of the object of nursing, we would be left with no proper end to direct our actions in nursing practice and, furthermore, to direct them in an ethical manner. Without the direction provided by ontological nursing knowledge, the end result of our efforts at inquiry would be chaos and, to use an apt phrase of Maritain's (1930), "a formless agglomeration" (p. 116).

Are there other kinds of philosophical nursing questions? I do not think so. I do not see a place for a derived nursing philosophy of man or of nature but instead hold that the principles of philosophy of man proper and of the philosophy of nature proper are taken on as assumption by nursing.

CONCLUDING REMARKS

During the last 2 decades, we have devoted much of our time and energy to the development of what has been called "the science of nursing." This devotion is misguided in that science cannot answer all of our questions. It is only by allowing philosophical inquiry to take its rightful place in nursing knowledge development that nurses stand a chance of not unknowingly violating the nursing profession, but rather of letting it be and become the powerful force that potentially lies in its nature to benefit humankind.

NOTE

1. This quote reflects the position taken by Adler (1965) with regard to the role of epistemology. However, it should be noted that when Adler made this statement, he was arguing that there is more to philosophy than epistemology—that philosophy addresses both first-order questions (i.e., "questions about that which is and happens or about what men should do and seek" [p. 44]) and second-order questions (i.e., "questions about our first-order knowledge, questions about the content of our thinking, when we try to answer first-order questions, or questions about the ways in which we express such thought in language" [p. 44]).

REFERENCES

Adler, M. J. (1965). *The conditions of philosophy*. New York: Atheneum.
Adler, M. J. (1985). *Ten philosophical mistakes*. New York: Macmillan.
Carper, B. (1975). *Fundamental patterns of knowing in nursing*. Unpublished doctoral dissertation, Columbia University, New York.
Chinn, P. L. (Ed.). (1989). Ethical issues [Special issue]. *Advances in Nursing Science, 11*(3).
Jacobs-Kramer, M. K., & Chinn, P. L. (1988). Perspectives on knowing: A model of nursing knowledge. *Scholarly Inquiry for Nursing Practice: An International Journal, 2*(2), 129-139.
Kidd, P., & Morrison, E. F. (1988). The progression of knowledge in nursing: A search for meaning. *Image, 20*(4). 222-224.

Maritain, J. (1930). *An introduction to philosophy* (E. I. Watkin, Trans.). London: Sheed & Ward.

Nicoll, L. H. (Ed.). (1986). *Perspectives on nursing theory.* Boston: Little, Brown.

Schlotfeldt, R. M. (1988). Structuring nursing knowledge: A priority for creating nursing's future. *Nursing Science Quarterly, 1*(1), 35-38.

Schultz, P. R., & Meleis, A. I. (1988). Nursing epistemology: Traditions, insights, questions. *Image, 20*(4), 217-221.

Walker, L. (1971). *Nursing as a discipline.* Unpublished doctoral dissertation, Indiana University, Indiana.

Wallace, W. A. (1977). *The elements of philosophy.* New York: Alba House.

3

The Aim of Philosophical Inquiry in Nursing: Unity or Diversity of Thought?

※

Perspective of SISTER M. SIMONE ROACH

Diversity always occurs in the light of new experience. Unity, on the other hand, has its basis in metaphysics. Unity is in the transcendent, the universal, rather than in the particular. It is found in first principles as, for example, in the frequently used principles: "The human person is worthy of respect" and "Do good; avoid evil or harm." With diversity there can also be unity, if we can hold to some primary or first principles.

In philosophical inquiry in nursing, is it not the case that we are searching for universal, transcendent principles when we attempt to conceptualize nursing and the many elements of a model or grand design? What is the meaning of *human*, or *human health*? What is the primary concept?

When I began to reflect on this challenging topic, I recalled the text of my first course in philosophy—*The Unity of Philosophical Experience* by Etienne Gilson (1937). Naturally, I was immediately

Author's Note: The writer acknowledges the contribution of Carol Opochinski, Department of Philosophy, University of Manitoba, for her comments on the first draft of this paper.

curious about what Gilson meant by unity. I would like to share some of his reflections.

According to Gilson, within the history of philosophy, there is evidence of some intrinsic intelligibility. There is a centuries-long experience of what philosophical knowledge is—and that such an experience exhibits a remarkable unity. This unity finds expression from Democritus, Plato, Aristotle, Plotinus, Christian philosophers, through Kant, Schopenhauer, Hegel, and Bergson, and through the 25 centuries of searching within the history of Western civilization, in the *necessity of first causes*. This is known as philosophy's *first law*.

The first law leads to the *second law*:

> By his very nature, man is a metaphysical animal. . . . There is, in human reason, a natural aptness, and consequently a natural urge, to transcend the limits of experience [to transcend the diversity] and to form transcendental notions by which the unity of knowledge may be completed. These are metaphysical notions. (pp. 307-308)[1]

The *third law* states, "Metaphysics is the knowledge gathered by a naturally transcendent reason in its search for first principles, or first causes, of what is given in sensible experience" (p. 308).[2]

In our search for first principles, we have not always reached our goal; oftentimes we have settled on a level of reductionist thinking. The problem of reductionism is encountered whenever we substitute concepts of any particular science, whether this be theology, logic, physics, biology, psychology, sociology, or economics, for those of metaphysics. These sciences are competent to solve their own problems. On the other hand, there is the *fourth law*: "As metaphysics aims at transcending all particular knowledge, no particular science is competent either to solve metaphysical problems or to judge their metaphysical solutions" (pp. 309-310).[3]

Gilson asserts that *being* is the first principle of all human knowledge; it is *a fortiori* the first principle of metaphysics. Metaphysics is the science[4] of being as being. Human thought is always about being:

> In the light of immediate evidence, the intellect sees that something is, or exists; that what exists is that which it is; that that which is, or exists, cannot be and not be at one and the same time;

that a thing either is, or it is not, and no third supposition is conceivable; last, but not least, that being only comes from being, which is the very root of the notion of causality. Reason has not to prove any one of these principles, otherwise they would not be principles, but conclusions; but it is by them that reason proves all the rest. (p. 314)[5]

What are the implications of these insights for nursing? Is there a metaphysics of nursing? Are there metaphysical principles, first principles that provide inspiration and that are the moving force, that is, the principles underlying all theories? I suggest a basis for unity in nursing thought, in two fundamental concepts: the concept of *human being* and the concept of *caring*.

Human reason is capable of uncovering the intrinsic meaning of human—the human being, as a metaphysical animal, as Gilson notes. In our diverse reflections, there is a thread of unity in the awareness of the mysterious, the sacred, the specialness, or uniqueness of the human being. We express this insight in some universal (transcendent) principles—a principle such as "the human being is worthy of respect." Is not this recognition a common (unified) center of gravitation for nursing theories or presuppositions?

However we might conceptualize nursing, we find nursing to subsume some notion of caring, of human care. That caring is central to nursing is a perception of nursing scholars and practitioners alike. How one approaches an inquiry into the nature of caring, however, is dictated by the nature of the questions asked. Questions may be on the level of ontology: "What is caring in itself?"; anthropology: "What does it mean to be a caring person?"; onticology: "What is a nurse doing when he or she is caring?"; epistemology: "How is caring known?"; and pedagogy: "How is caring learned and taught?" (Roach, 1984, 1987).

In the early stages of my research on caring, I focused on the ontic level, coming up with statements that were attributional and specific. I categorized these statements under the *five Cs:* compassion, competence, confidence, conscience, and commitment.

This early research, however, left a disturbing void that I (as a "metaphysical animal") was trying to fill. I was searching for unity, that is, an ontology of caring rather than a diversity of attributes that these ontic statements provided.

Finally, the leap occurred and I discovered something intrinsic to my being as a human person, not as nurse, but as a human person, an insight that I suggest flows from an anthropological vision. This insight became the basis for a further conceptualization of caring as central to nursing. The following are its key elements:

- Caring is the human mode of being.
- I care, not because I am a nurse, but because I am a human being.
- Nursing is the professionalization of the human capacity to care, through the acquisition and use of the knowledge and skill required for prescribed nursing roles.
- Caring is not unique *to* nursing in that it distinguishes nursing from other professions or avocations; rather, caring is unique *in* nursing in that of all the concepts used to describe nursing, caring is unique. Caring is a universal (transcendent) concept that subsumes all others.
- Nursing does not differ from other helping professions in that it cares, but it differs in the manner in which it cares, within prescribed roles, using a discrete body of knowledge and skill (Roach, 1984, 1987).

SOME THOUGHTS TOWARD A SYNTHESIS

In reflections on nursing, there exists, at certain levels, diversity of thought. This diversity is evident in various theoretical formulations despite their common elements. Unity exists in the universal insights that have captured the imagination of nurse practitioners as well as those of nurse scientists, and is evident from the beginning of nursing's recorded history.

To paraphrase Gilson's reflections on philosophy, in relation to nursing, there is evidence of some "intrinsic intelligibility" in the history of nursing. From the earliest records of human history, there is evidence of human care and of a moral consciousness, however primitive, of the duty to care. In retrospect, this may be interpreted as a natural human urge or response. Loren Eiseley (1960), an anthropologist, offers an example that seems to affirm this insight.

Forty thousand years ago in the bleak uplands of southwestern Asia, a man, a Neanderthal man, once labeled by the Darwinian proponents of struggle as a ferocious ancestral beast—a man whose face might cause you some slight uneasiness if he sat beside you— a man of this sort existed with a fearful body handicap in that ice-age world. He had lost an arm. But still he lived and was cared for. Somebody, some group of human things, in a hard, violent

and stony world, loved this maimed creature enough to cherish
him. (pp. 144-145)[6]

The following commentary by Maguire (1978) offers further insights on Eiseley's reflections:

> Somewhere back there in the period of harsh beginnings, there
> appeared, in Eiseley's words, loving, caring and cherishing. Con-
> cern was born and with it, morality. Eiseley compares its emer-
> gence to "a faint light, like a patch of sunlight moving over the
> dark shadows on a forest floor." What it was was the light of a
> distinctively human consciousness, animated by the unique en-
> ergy that we have come to call love. This capacity for love, this
> ability to appreciate and respond to the value of personal life in
> all its forms, is the foundation of moral consciousness. The ap-
> pearance of this capacity was an event more significant for human
> existence than the first appearances of technology or of art, al-
> though these latter events are more easily chronicled and have
> won more attention. Yet somewhere back there, the signs of moral-
> value-consciousness appear. It might be visible, for example, in
> the ceremonial burying of the dead which began before the extinc-
> tion of Neanderthal man. Along with ever-present superstition,
> the liturgies of burial could be a sign of grief, and thus of concern
> and love. More to the point is Arnold Toynbee's observation that
> "the distinction between good and evil seems to have been drawn
> by all human beings at all times and places. The drawing of it
> seems, in fact, to be one of the intrinsic and universal characteris-
> tics of our common nature." (p. 86)[7]

This common thread, evident in the early history of the human
race and indeed in the history of nursing, as a human response to
human need, has also characterized nursing developments to the
present. The focal points of human care, human person, and person-in-relation (the human community), along with a duty to care,
mark the unifying elements and the ground for "first causes" or
"first principles" in nursing.

We have had our share of reductionism in nursing, more evident
in nursing education whenever undue weight has been given to
science or a science. Any one science, or science as a whole, is limited to a particular area of competence. Science cannot ask, let alone
answer, all the questions pertaining to human beings, life, and
living. Because of a slanted reductionism, we have occasionally

found ourselves in contradiction with our own premises—promoting a holistic conceptualization of nursing within a decidedly reductionist or fragmented anthropology. Unity has its basis in metaphysics. Without metaphysics, nursing loses its moorings. A metaphysics provides nursing with the source of its unity, the basis for

an anthropological vision that is holistic: the human being is a body-mind-spirit unity rather than a sum of parts, a metaphysical being capable of grasping transcendent principles;

a vision of caring that is an expression of the intrinsically human caring as the human mode of being;

a vision of education that presupposes an integral, holistic humanism, which acknowledges mind-body-spirit unity and the universe of knowledge that contributes to and is required for human understanding; and

a vision of the human person as person-in-relation (the notion of human community), of human moral awareness with ethical-moral bonds.

NOTES

1. Reprinted with permission of Charles Scribner's Sons, an imprint of Macmillan Publishing Company, from *The Unity of Philosophical Experience* (pp. 307-310, 314) by Etienne Gilson. Copyright © 1937 by Charles Scribner's Sons; copyright renewed © 1965 by Etienne Gilson.
2. Reprinted with permission of Charles Scribner's Sons, an imprint of Macmillan Publishing Company, from *The Unity of Philosophical Experience* (pp. 307-310, 314) by Etienne Gilson. Copyright © 1937 by Charles Scribner's Sons; copyright renewed © 1965 by Etienne Gilson.
3. Reprinted with permission of Charles Scribner's Sons, an imprint of Macmillan Publishing Company, from *The Unity of Philosophical Experience* (pp. 307-310, 314) by Etienne Gilson. Copyright © 1937 by Charles Scribner's Sons; copyright renewed © 1965 by Etienne Gilson.
4. *Science* is here used in the classical sense, meaning *knowledge*.
5. Reprinted with permission of Charles Scribner's Sons, an imprint of Macmillan Publishing Company, from *The Unity of Philosophical Experience* (pp. 307-310, 314) by Etienne Gilson. Copyright © 1937 by Charles Scribner's Sons; copyright renewed © 1965 by Etienne Gilson.
6. Reprinted with permission of Atheneum Publishers, an imprint of Macmillan Publishing Company, from *The Firmament of Time* (pp. 144-145) by Loren Eiseley. Copyright © 1960 by Loren Eiseley; copyright © 1960 by the trustees of the University of Pennsylvania.
7. Reprinted with permission of Doubleday, from *The Moral Choice* (p. 86) by Daniel Maguire. Copyright © 1978 by Doubleday.

REFERENCES

Eiseley, L. (1960). *The firmament of time*. New York: Atheneum.
Gilson, E. (1937). *The unity of philosophical experience*. New York: Scribner.
Maguire, D. (1978). *The moral choice*. New York: Doubleday.
Roach, M. S. (1984). *Caring, the human mode of being: Implications for nursing*. Toronto: University of Toronto, Faculty of Nursing.
Roach, M. S. (1987). *The human act of caring. Blueprint for the health professions*. Ottawa: Canadian Hospital Association.

4

The Aim of Philosophical Inquiry in Nursing: Unity or Diversity of Thought?

✳

Perspective of JOHN R. PHILLIPS

Nursing is in the process of creating a science of nursing in service to humankind. Without an understanding of philosophy in nursing, there can be no science of nursing. This is especially true because philosophy is the science of all sciences (Runes, 1960). Philosophical inquiry in nursing enables one to criticize and systematize nursing knowledge that has been gleaned from empirical research, clinical practice, rational learning, or any other source of knowledge, including intuitive knowing.

Philosophy is especially significant in nursing, because both deal with the humanistic aspects of life. Philosophy enables nursing to focus on characteristics of human beings and their potentials as they experience their realities. Through use of this knowledge, nurses can help people to gain understanding of their relationship with the environment to achieve optimum health.

Philosophical inquiry brings unity to the diversity of thought in nursing. This is especially true when one considers Polanyi's (1964) "tacit knowing" and "explicit knowing." The bringing into awareness of tacit knowing, through philosophical inquiry, is significant because it is a valid way to help create a science of nursing. Once this way of knowing is understood, it can be communicated through explicit knowing. The integral nature of this process provides unity to ways of knowing to get at the wholeness of phenomena central to nursing.

Such knowledge attainment in nursing calls for a philosophical vision (Burnham & Wheelwright, 1932), which requires nurses' willingness to understand and appreciate the diversity of thought in nursing. Through philosophical inquiry, nurses move beyond stereotypical and narrow perceptions of nursing and scientific inquiry to perceive the wholeness of nursing. This provides understanding of the hidden, actual, and alternative meanings in the diverse views of nursing. This moves nurses to holistic understanding whereby both the potentials and limitations of each nursing view are comprehended.

The evolution of this unity in diversity of thought in nursing provides new doors of perception that go beyond the visible human condition to an understanding of the ground of the becoming of human beings. New insight into what it means to be human arises. Thus, the discovery of the philosophy integral to the science of nursing brings an understanding that contributes to unity in diversity of thought in nursing.

Philosophical inquiry brings to the forefront an undivided wholeness whereby nursing can elucidate the philosophical foundation for its diverse nursing models (Sarter, 1988). Our current philosophical inquiry makes manifest the knowledge used to systematize nursing models and the validity of the knowledge generated through use of the models. This inquiry clarifies the structure and meaning relevant to each nursing model. In the process, there is a disclosure of the ambiguities and inconsistencies in nurses' thinking about the models, especially because there is a revealing of the philosophical assumptions of each model. Relevant distinctions of each model are identified so one can draw consistent conclusions about each nursing model and its knowledge, language, and reality.

Philosophical inquiry enables one to go beyond the current reductionistic, mechanistic analysis of nursing models to get at the wholeness of nursing. If nursing science is to advance through use of its nursing models, nurses can no longer be hypnotized by the traditional scientific methods and modes of analysis. Nursing must move toward forms of philosophical inquiry that get at the philosophical themes of the wholeness of nursing. Philosophical inquiry must be seen as a scientific method that can be used to investigate phenomena of nursing that are not well understood by any science (Manchester, 1986).

Our current methods of philosophical inquiry and nursing models are attempts to get at the hidden significant aspects of humans experiencing their realities. Yet, there is a wholeness of the science of nursing that is not manifest in the sum of the knowledge of each nursing model. A holistic view departs from the reductionistic belief that the wholeness of nursing science can be understood from knowledge of the individual nursing models (Harman, 1988; Rogers, 1970).

This holistic view enables one to peer into an indivisible whole similar to Bohm's (1980) implicate order.[1] The implicate order of wholeness of nursing science enfolds the philosophical themes common to all nursing models. Our current nursing science, as manifest in nursing models and their theories, is an explicate unfolding of this larger philosophical implicate order. As nurses continue to unfold this implicate philosophical nursing order, there will be greater understanding of nursing models to further enhance unity in diversity of nursing thought.

The philosophical implicate order of nursing science becomes important when one considers Bronowski's (1965) statement that "all science is a search for unity and hidden likenesses" (p. 15). This search has involved a gradual unfolding of the implicate wholeness of nursing. This is evidenced in the early nursing literature, which is replete with concepts drawn from other sciences. These views helped nurses to understand people primarily from a disease perspective. This fragmentary view was not effective in understanding the wholeness of people.

Some early nursing theorists, recognizing the limitations of the medical model, chose concepts that were relevant to the process of nursing, those that focused on its caring aspects. In this respect, theorists such as Peplau (1952), Wiedenbach (1964), Rogers (1961, 1964), and Henderson (1966) signify an early concern for the whole person and for a philosophical foundation for nursing. Nurse theorists continued to develop nursing models, and they were explicit in showing how the concepts were related to each other. Specific assumptions of the models were stated, many of them based in philosophy.

Fawcett (1989) has presented a metaparadigm of nursing in an attempt to give unity in the diversity of nursing models. The proposed relationships among the metaparadigm concepts are flavored with philosophy and are in need of further philosophical explication. Fawcett also delineates the various nursing models into categories such as developmental, systems, or interaction in an attempt to give unity to them.

Parse (1987) has presented the totality and the simultaneity paradigms that get more at the philosophical differences among the various nursing models. These two paradigms make a distinction in how people are viewed as parts and as a whole. However, it is only of late that nursing has begun to look for the philosophical foundations common to nursing models (Sarter, 1988). Sarter points out that a metaparadigm is needed that supports a variety of nursing models, "while maintaining a coherent and common philosophical orientation" (p. 52). Inquiry into the philosophical nature of nursing models helps nurses to move beyond discussing the facts and concepts of the models to perceive the models as a whole.

The integral nature of philosophical inquiry avoids splitting up the phenomena of nursing into subjective or objective. As such, it is concerned with a "wholeness" rather than a "parts" perspective. If philosophical inquiry is concerned with the unitary nature of phenomena, then the concept of prime importance, of which Sarter (1988) speaks, will be *pattern*. Newman (1986) states, "The pattern is in information that depicts the whole understanding of the meaning of all the relationships at once. It is a fundamental attribute of all there is and gives unity in diversity" (p. 13). From a qualitative perspective, philosophical inquiry can be used to discover underlying dimensions and patterns of relationships found in nursing science. Pattern seeing brings together facts and ideas into a coherent whole. Of significance here is Carper's (1978) patterns of knowing in nursing. An understanding of these patterns increases awareness of the unity in diversity of nursing knowledge. Philosophical inquiry confirms that wholeness of nursing, and people, involves mutual pattern changes rather than the mechanistic process of cause and effect and adaptation. In fact, there is a need for philosophical inquiry into how change in phenomena is represented in the various nursing models. It is these pattern changes that are manifestations of the philosophical implicate order of wholeness of nursing science. Recognition of these patterns changes the way nurses think about phenomena; in fact, they will see phenomena that were present but were not seen before.

Philosophical inquiry will bring unity to nursing through a clarification of nursing diagnosis, if that concept is retained in the nursing nomenclature of the future. Currently, many of the nursing diagnoses retain a parts, disease, or medical orientation. This will change as philosophical inquiry refines the meaning of the concepts of nursing science to enhance pattern seeing. Once this happens, nursing care will be based on pattern diagnosing rather than on parts or disease diagnosing. The current NANDA list of nursing diagnoses is reflective of this beginning change.

Thus, the aim of philosophical inquiry in nursing is unity in diversity of thought. Ellis (1983) states clearly that all nursing theory or research derives from or leads to philosophy. Philosophical inquiry enhances seeing all phenomena as wholes. The development of philosophical themes gives insight into the patterns of the implicate order of nursing science. We can no longer afford to let traditional science impede the unfolding of nursing science through restrictions placed on pattern seeing.

As Harman (1988) said, "Perhaps the time has come to tiptoe no longer, but to quietly, firmly, and self-confidently insist on the need for a restructuring of science to accommodate all, rather than just part, of human experience" (p. 21). We have only begun to understand the implicate wholeness of nursing science. Philosophical inquiry fosters creative change, the seeking for discovery of knowledge to expand nursing science. It will be philosophical inquiry that unfolds knowledge that brings greater unity in diversity of thought in nursing. Ultimately, philosophical inquiry enables nursing to achieve its goal of care for the whole person. The core of nursing lies in the wholeness of human beings.

NOTE

1. Bohm (1980) sees the universe as indivisible, a flowing unbroken wholeness; everything is interconnected. The implicate order of this wholeness means "everything is enfolded into everything" (p. 177), whereby space and time are no longer the dominant factors to determine the relationships of different elements. The movement of the whole expresses itself through explicate forms whereby parts are manifestations of Bohm's flowing wholeness, the deeper implicate order. In the explicate order, things are unfolded whereby "each thing lies only in its own particular region of space (and time) and outside the regions belonging to other things" (p. 177).

REFERENCES

Bohm, D. (1980). *Wholeness and the implicate order*. London: Routledge & Kegan Paul.

Bronowski, J. (1965). *Science and human values*. New York: Harper & Row.

Burnham, J., & Wheelwright, P. (1932). *Introduction to philosophical analysis*. New York: Holt, Rinehart & Winston.

Carper, B. A. (1978). Fundamental patterns of knowing in nursing. *Advances in Nursing Science, 1*(1), 13-23.

Ellis, R. (1983). Philosophic inquiry. In H. H. Werley & J. J. Fitzpatrick (Eds.), *Annual review of nursing research* (Vol. 1, pp. 211-228). New York: Springer.

Fawcett, J. (1989). *Analysis and evaluation of conceptual models of nursing* (2nd ed.). Philadelphia: Davis.

Harman, W. W. (1988). The transpersonal challenge to the scientific paradigm: The need for a restructuring of science. *Revision, 11*(2), 13-21.

Henderson, V. (1966). *The nature of nursing: A definition and its implications, practice, research, and education*. New York: Macmillan.

Manchester, P. (1986). Analytic philosophy and foundational inquiry: The method. In P. L. Munhall & C. J. Oiler (Eds.), *Nursing research: A qualitative perspective* (pp. 229-249). New York: Appleton-Century-Crofts.

Newman, M. A. (1986). *Health as expanding consciousness*. St. Louis: C. V. Mosby.

Parse, R. (1987). *Nursing science: Major paradigms, theories, and critiques*. Philadelphia: W. B. Saunders.

Peplau, H. E. (1952). *Interpersonal relations in nursing*. New York: Putnam.

Polanyi, M. (1964). *Personal knowledge: Toward a post-critical philosophy*. New York: Harper Torchbooks.

Rogers, M. E. (1961). *Educational revolution in nursing*. New York: Macmillan.

Rogers, M. E. (1964). *Reveille in nursing*. Philadelphia: Davis.

Rogers, M. E. (1970). *An introduction to the theoretical basis of nursing*. Philadelphia: Davis.

Runes, D. D. (Ed.). (1960). *Dictionary of philosophy* (15th ed. rev.). New York: Philosophical Library.

Sarter, B. (1988). Philosophical sources of nursing theory. *Nursing Science Quarterly, 1*(2), 52-59.

Wiedenbach, E. (1964). *Clinical nursing: A helping art*. New York: Springer.

PART TWO

The Place of Philosophic
Inquiry in Nursing

The potential contribution to the nurse's world of the application of philosophic inquiry in nursing has in large part gone unrecognized. To understand the nature of philosophic inquiry in nursing is one thing; to understand its significance is another. The latter is grounded in the former. To understand the potential for good that lies within an entity requires an understanding of the capacities, the nature, of that entity.

Were more nurse researchers to become cognizant of the potential that lies within philosophic inquiry to advance the discipline of nursing, surely they would embrace it. Who would refuse to invite into our research endeavors that which would shed light on and help us out of the many epistemological entanglements in which we find ourselves? However, if we do not ground its application in an understanding of that which it can legitimately contribute to the discipline by virtue of its special capacities, then we are in danger of exchanging unrecognized potential for unrealized potential.

The intention behind the inclusions of Part Two is to goad readers into philosophizing about the place of philosophic inquiry in nursing. In reading these three essays, readers might ask themselves the following questions: What place or role is philosophic inquiry accorded? What place or role ought it to be accorded? In other words, of what use is philosophic inquiry in nursing?

Carper's essay (Chapter 7), describing her seminal work on the fundamental patterns of knowing in nursing, provides a notable example of the place accorded philosophic inquiry in nursing by some nurse researchers. In their essays, Adam (Chapter 5) and Fawcett (Chapter 6) tackle the difficult philosophic issue of whether contemporary conceptualizations of nursing are philosophy or science. In large part, their treatment of this issue leaves open the question of the place of philosophic nursing inquiry in relation to these conceptualizations. But because the issue is a philosophic (not a scientific) one, it would seem that its final resolution is dependent upon philosophic inquiry in nursing being accorded some place in future nursing endeavors. The questions that follow are designed, in part, to help readers to identify what this place ought to be.

Guiding Questions: Making Up Your Own Mind

1. Is philosophic inquiry in nursing all or largely critical and analytic of existing knowledge, or does it stand to give us knowledge of what is and happens in the nurse's world?

2. Does philosophic nursing knowledge in any way govern scientific nursing knowledge?

3. What is the relationship of contemporary conceptualizations of nursing to the structure of nursing knowledge?

4. If the empirical test of truth is seen to be applicable to the products of both scientific and philosophic nursing inquiry, does it also apply to contemporary conceptualizations of nursing?

5. What are the relationships among scientific nursing theories, philosophic nursing theories, and contemporary conceptualizations of nursing?

5

Contemporary Conceptualizations of Nursing: Philosophy or Science?

✳

Perspective of EVELYN ADAM

By contemporary conceptualizations of nursing, I understand conceptualizations that are specific to nursing, that is, those conceptions created by nurses for nursing and that are sufficiently explicit as to be known as conceptual models for nursing. I must make a point of this, because one of the more popular contemporary conceptualizations of nursing is borrowed from medicine; others have been borrowed from psychology, ecology, and sociology (Phillips, 1977/1986). In this paper, then, only those conceptions of nursing that are known as conceptual models for nursing will be considered.

Are the contemporary conceptions of nursing philosophies? Let us first look at what constitutes a philosophy. Philosophy is concerned with (among other things) the nature of being, the nature of reality, the purpose of human life, and the limits of knowledge (Silva, 1977/1986). Two philosophers well-known to nurses, Dickoff and James (1970), define philosophy as a set of mind or as a habitual approach.

Curtin (1979) discusses the philosophical foundations of nursing; she maintains that the essence of nursing is the nurse-patient relationship in which the nurse ideally has a humanizing

influence on patient care and recognizes human rights and needs.[1]
Curtin's humanistic philosophy is evident.

Other philosophies are also espoused by nurse authors, and I
am indebted to graduate students at the University of Arizona
(Holecek & Kane, 1971) for the following condensed version of
some of them:

- Socratic—know thyself
- Realism—be thyself
- Humanism—give thyself
- Rationalism—understand thyself
- Naturalism—describe thyself
- Pragmatism—prove thyself
- Idealism—imagine thyself
- Existentialism—choose thyself

Nurse authors, who discuss the caring relationship, humanistic
values, moral beliefs, patient participation, holism, and the therapeutic use of self, seem to reveal underlying idealistic and humanistic philosophies. Nurse authors who stress problem-solving and
scientific principles and who argue that nursing is an art and a
science seem to reveal rationalistic and pragmatic tendencies.

Nurses, as indeed all health professionals, may have a mind set
that is idealistic and humanistic and, at the same time, pragmatic.
Nurses, as indeed other health professionals, may have a habitual
approach that seems to be rationalistic as well as existentialist. A
nurse's underlying philosophy gives important direction to her
life. It is, however, concerned with the nature of being, not the nature of nursing. It deals with the purpose of human life, not the
purpose of nursing. A frame of reference at a lower level of abstraction is necessary to guide a professional discipline's research,
practice, and education. That frame of reference is a conceptual
model for nursing: a contemporary conceptualization of nursing.

An important part of a conceptual model is its assumptions, and
the importance given to them may be due to an underlying rationalism; Roy's (1984) assumptions, for example, are drawn largely
from Helson's adaptation-level theory whereas Johnson's (1980) are
drawn from general systems theory. The beliefs and values, also an
important part of a conceptual model, are, on the whole, idealistic

and humanistic; the authors of conceptual models for nursing make clear their belief in the social importance of nursing and in the distinctiveness of nursing's service to humanity. The goal of nursing, the first major unit of a conceptual model, can be considered idealistic, pragmatic, and humanistic. Independence in need satisfaction (Henderson, 1966) and behavioral equilibrium (Johnson, 1980) are examples. The conceptualization of the client, the second major unit, is surely existential and humanistic. It is also holistic, another mind-set or habitual approach. Consider Roy's four adaptive modes (1984), Henderson's fourteen basic needs (1966), Orem's eight activities known as self-care (1985), and Johnson's seven behavioral subsystems (1980). The social role of the nurse, the third major unit, is very often humanistic and idealistic. The source of difficulty, the fourth major unit, seems to be highly pragmatic because it defines the parameters of the nurse's jurisdiction. The fifth and sixth major units, the intervention and the desired consequences, may be seen as indicative of a humanistic, idealistic, and pragmatic approach.

The models reveal philosophical foundations; they contain some philosophical statements. But a few philosophical statements do not a philosophy make. The models are not philosophies; they are conceptual models. I am aware that the contemporary conceptualizations of nursing are often referred to as philosophies. I have heard people speak of Johnson's philosophy or of Henderson's philosophy. Those conceptions of nursing are not philosophies. They do not consider the purpose and nature of life and being but the purpose and nature of one discipline: nursing. They reveal holistic foundations, they demonstrate idealistic attitudes, they present pragmatic mind sets, but they are not philosophies, and in my opinion no apology should ever be made for that fact.

Are the contemporary conceptualizations of nursing a science? Science has been defined as a systematic body of knowledge (Dessler, cited in Gruending, 1985); as a consensual, informed opinion about the natural world, rather than a body of codified knowledge (Gortner & Schultz, 1988); and as a process of knowing and challenging (Newman, 1983). For Greene (1979), science is both a process (the scientific method) and a body of organized knowledge (rather than intuitive or common knowledge). Discussing the philosophies of science, Silva and Rothbart (1984) point out that logical empiricists conceive of science only in terms of the results (the product) whereas historicists understand science as a process of human behaviour and thought.

Whatever the definition of science that is accepted, the question that is frequently asked is "Is nursing a science?" At this conference, the question is rather, "Are the conceptions of nursing a science?" The question could have been "Are contemporary conceptions of nursing, theories?" because, for those who see science as a systematic body of knowledge, the tool of science is research and the major expression of science is theory. Rather than examining the various definitions of theory, I will remind you of the one offered by Roy and Roberts (1981): "a system of interrelated propositions used to describe, predict, explain, understand, and control a part of the empirical world" (p. 5).

Contemporary conceptualizations of nursing certainly have scientific and theoretical components. The assumptions of a conceptual model are drawn from two sources: clinical and theoretical. Consider the theoretical sources of the Henderson, Roy, and Johnson models; they are, respectively, Thorndike's theory, Helson's theory, and general systems theory. The major units of the models are logically derived from those assumptions. It is therefore reasonable to state that the current conceptual models for nursing have a theoretical or scientific base; that base can, of course, always be contested. However, some scientific underpinnings do not a science make. The fact that a conceptual model has a sound theoretical foundation does not make it any less a conceptual model; a solid theoretical base does not turn a model into a theory. A conceptual model is not made up of propositions to be validated, nor is it composed of hypotheses to be tested (Adam, 1987). Fawcett (1978) has pointed out that conceptual models cannot be empirically tested because of the abstract nature of their concepts.

The truth element, which is associated with both philosophy and science, is not an intrinsic part of a conceptual model. In as much as a conceptual model for nursing indicates that discipline's focus of scientific inquiry, it is the departure point for research and the seeking of truth; of itself, the model cannot be considered true or untrue, right or wrong (Johnson, 1974). The model is a way of conceptualizing nursing; it is a nursing perspective. If it proves to be socially useful, congruent, and significant (Johnson, 1974), it will lead to the discovery of truth in those matters that are of scientific concern to nursing. For example, researchers working from Henderson's perspective might, in the process of knowing and of challenging, develop a body of codified understanding of client independence in need satisfaction. They would be truth-seeking developers of nursing science, the expression of which might be a theory of client independence, a theory of complementing client knowledge, or a theory of supplementing client motivation. Researchers working from another frame of reference for nursing would develop theories about quite different phenomena. If the knowledge generated by one group of researchers proved to be in conflict with that developed by another group, more research would be stimulated and the science of nursing would be further advanced (Adam, 1987). It is my opinion that nursing theories can be developed only from a nursing perspective, that nursing science can be advanced only from a nursing frame of reference, and that research is nursing research only if it examines phenomena of specific interest to nursing, that is, phenomena that are indicated by one or the other of the conceptual models for nursing.

Contemporary conceptualizations of nursing: philosophy or science? They are neither. They are ways of conceptualizing our discipline and, as such, should be recognized for what they are: conceptual models for nursing. Trying to see them as something that they are not is, to my mind, another case of the "emperor's clothes."

The current conceptualizations of nursing have been presented for many years as the conceptual base for nursing research, practice, and education. Phillips (1977/1986) makes a strong case for conceptual models in the advancement of nursing science. Roy and Roberts (1981) are of the opinion that most master's degree programs in nursing have courses explaining conceptual models and that, in some places, the student's thesis research must be drawn from one of the existing models. Yet conceptual models for nursing are often referred to as macrotheories, are frequently considered to be untested theories, and at times are even seen as a serious threat to nursing.

Conceptual models must of course be evaluated. They cannot be tested or validated as though they were theories but can and should be evaluated. A conceptual model should be criticized, and perhaps condemned outright, if it does not meet the intrinsic criteria of clarity, consistency, and completeness. A model must also meet the extrinsic criteria of social utility, significance, and congruence (Johnson, 1974). However, the criticism directed toward conceptual models is often indicative of a lack of understanding of what the conceptual basis of a professional discipline really is.

Conceptual models have, for example, been criticized for not dealing adequately with the phenomenon of death (Hoon, 1986); it is argued that, because death is an important part of life, the models should include death as one of their concepts. I must reject that criticism, because the same argument could be made for other important stages of life: aging, adolescence, early childhood, and so forth. It seems to negate the fact that the models are conceptualizations of *nursing*, whatever the stage of development of a particular client. Models were never intended to include every concept of interest to nursing; the nurse who is particularly interested in touch, or in pain, will certainly not find her favorite concept mentioned in a conceptual model for the nursing profession.

Models have also been taken to task for being rigid and inflexible (Hardy, 1986) and therefore potentially unfair to consumers. The so-called unfairness is illustrated in the following "dangerous" situation: A nurse who adhered to a developmental model might seek to impose it on a consumer, who, if he were an engineer, would be following a systems model; because of the lesser power wielded by the consumer, he could not win. It is my opinion that such arguments lose sight of an important consideration: an engineer seeking help from a professional nurse has every right to expect that the nurse have a clear conception of his/her service to society; when the nurse requests the help of a professional engineer, the nurse will expect him/her to have an engineering frame of reference, a clear conception of his/her service to society.

Conceptualizations of nursing have been criticized for their high degree of abstraction and for their dangerous professionalizing ambitions. Lundh, Soder, and Waerness (1988) refer to the conceptions as nursing theories, pointing out that a nursing theory is a description of two things: the nursing process and the system in which nursing takes place. I find it difficult to accept that definition of nursing theory; the nursing process is merely a systematic method, and the system in which nursing takes place is hardly a conception of nursing. The degree of abstraction of conceptual models is precisely what permits their usefulness, whatever the context in which the nurse finds herself, be it hospital nursing, community nursing, education, or research.

Many nurses view the contemporary conceptualizations of nursing as interesting material for academic discussions but not quite worthy of their confidence as a conceptual base for choosing a research problem, organizing a curriculum, or planning nursing care. In a given situation, those nurses prefer to base their actions on specific knowledge that they have acquired: principles of administration, the helping relationship, alternative treatment modalities, family dynamics, and so forth. Instead of seeing that same knowledge as particularly useful to them in the pursuit of their professional goal (as indicated by a conceptual model for nursing), they seem to consider the knowledge an *alternative* to a nursing perspective. In another situation, those nurses turn to other existing knowledge. They remain curiously reluctant to adopt a conceptual model that would encourage them to make use of that same knowledge in order to attain a goal broad enough to encompass all nursing activities.

The state of understanding of conceptions of nursing was illustrated in the United States as recently as 1987, in a national survey of nurse respondents who had either master's or doctoral preparation (Jacobson, 1987). Many questions received positive and encouraging answers. However, when asked to identify the "conceptual models of nursing" with which they were familiar, many respondents named the following: Selye's stress model, Piaget's work, general systems theory, problem solving, and Maslow's hierarchy of needs. To quote Alice: "Curiouser and curiouser!" If the survey had been conducted in Canada, the answers to that question might have been even more embarrassing. It seems that even well-prepared nurses understand "conceptual models of nursing" to be any framework that, at one time or another, is useful to a nurse.

I have attempted to establish that a contemporary conceptualization of nursing is neither philosophy nor science. It is an entity in its own right with its own name: conceptual model for nursing. It is the cornerstone of nursing's development. In closing, I leave you with one of my favorite quotes, from the first issue of *Advances in Nursing Science:* "It is the general conception of any field of inquiry that ultimately determines the kind of knowledge the field aims to develop as well as the manner in which that knowledge is to be organized, tested and applied" (Carper, 1978, p. 13).

62 THE PLACE OF INQUIRY

NOTE

1. The same author refers to "models of nursing" (p. 2) as the nurse as caretaker, the nurse as health educator, the nurse as physician assistant, and so forth.

REFERENCES

1. The same author refers to "models of nursing" (p. 2) as the nurse as caretaker, the nurse as health educator, the nurse as physician assistant, and so forth.

Adam, E. (1987). Nursing theory: What it is and what it is not. *Nursing Papers, 19*(1), 5-14.

Carper, B. (1978). Fundamental patterns of knowing in nursing. *Advances in Nursing Science, 1*(1), 13-23.

Curtin, L. L. (1979). The nurse as advocate: A philosophical foundation for nursing. *Advances in Nursing Science, 1*(3), 1-10.

Dickoff, J., & James, P. (1970). Beliefs and values: Bases for curriculum design. *Nursing Research, 19*(5), 415-427.

Fawcett, J. (1978). The relationship between theory and research: A double helix. *Advances in Nursing Science, 1*(1), 49-62.

Gortner, S. R., & Schultz, P. R. (1988). Approaches to nursing science methods. *Image, 20*(1), 22-24.

Greene, J. A. (1979). Science, nursing and nursing science: A conceptual analysis. *Advances in Nursing Science, 2*(1), 57-64.

Gruending, D. L. (1985). Nursing theory: A vehicle of professionalization? *Journal of Advanced Nursing, 10*, 553-558.

Hardy, L. K. (1986). (Janforum). Identifying the place of theoretical frameworks in an evolving discipline. *Journal of Advanced Nursing, 11*, 103-107.

Henderson, V. (1966). *The nature of nursing*. New York: Macmillan.

Holecek, M. F., & Kane, S. C. (1971). (Incoming mail). *Nursing Research, 20*(5), 459.

Hoon, E. (1986). Game playing: A way to look at nursing models. *Journal of Advanced Nursing, 11*, 421-427.

Jacobson, S. F. (1987). Studying and using conceptual models of nursing. *Image, 19*(2), 78-82.

Johnson, D. E. (1974). Development of theory: A requisite for nursing as a primary health profession. *Nursing Research, 23*(5), 372-377.

Johnson, D. E. (1980). The behavioral system model for nursing. In J. P. Riehl & C. Roy (Eds.), *Conceptual models for nursing practice* (2nd ed., pp. 207-216). New York: Appleton-Century-Crofts.

Lundh, U., Soder, M., & Waerness, K. (1988). Nursing theories: A critical view. *Image, 20*(1), 36-40.

Newman, M. A. (1983). The continuing revolution: A history of nursing science. In N. L. Chaska (Ed.), *The nursing profession: A time to speak* (pp. 385-393). New York: McGraw-Hill.

Orem, D. E. (1985). *Nursing: Concepts of practice* (3rd ed.). New York: McGraw-Hill.

Phillips, J. R. (1986). Nursing systems and nursing models. In L. H. Nicoll (Ed.), *Perspectives on nursing theory* (pp. 354-358). Boston: Little, Brown. (Reprinted from *Image, 9*(1), pp. 4-7, 1977)

Roy, C. (1984). *Introduction to nursing: An adaptation model* (2nd ed.). Englewood Cliffs, NJ: Prentice-Hall.

Roy, C., & Roberts, S. L. (1981). *Theory construction in nursing: An adaptation model.* Englewood Cliffs, NJ: Prentice-Hall.

Silva, M. C. (1986). Philosophy, science, theory: Interrelationships and implications for nursing research. In L. H. Nicoll (Ed.), *Perspectives on nursing theory* (pp. 563-568). Boston: Little, Brown. (Reprinted from *Image, 9*(3), pp. 59-63, 1977)

Silva, M. C., & Rothbart, D. (1984). An analysis of changing trends in philosophies of science on nursing theory development and testing. *Advances in Nursing Science, 6*(2), 1-13.

6

Contemporary Conceptualizations of Nursing: Philosophy or Science?

✳

Perspective of JACQUELINE FAWCETT

My response to the panel topic "Contemporary Conceptualizations of Nursing: Philosophy or Science?" is based on my view of the structural hierarchy of contemporary nursing knowledge. Collectively, the structural hierarchy encompasses the current conceptualizations of nursing. The hierarchy is illustrated in Figure 6.1.

THE METAPARADIGM

The first, and most abstract and general, component of the structural hierarchy of nursing knowledge is what Thomas Kuhn (1977) called the *metaparadigm*. A metaparadigm is the most global perspective of a discipline and "acts as an encapsulating unit, or framework, within which the more restricted . . . structures develop" (Eckberg & Hill, 1979, p. 927). A metaparadigm identifies certain phenomena that are of interest to a discipline

---

Author's Note: Portions of this paper are adapted with permission of F. A. Davis, from *Analysis and Evaluation of Conceptual Models of Nursing* (2nd ed.) by J. Fawcett. Copyright © 1989 by F. A. Davis.

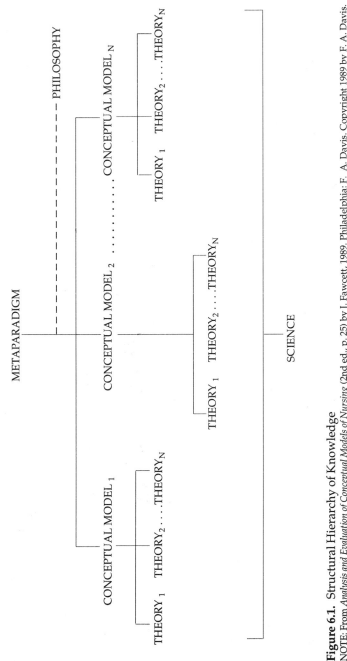

Figure 6.1. Structural Hierarchy of Knowledge

NOTE: From *Analysis and Evaluation of Conceptual Models of Nursing* (2nd ed., p. 25) by J. Fawcett, 1989. Philadelphia: F. A. Davis. Copyright 1989 by F. A. Davis. Adapted by permission.

and explains how that discipline deals with those phenomena in an unique manner.

Metaparadigm of Nursing

Considerable agreement now exists that the central concepts of the metaparadigm of nursing are person, environment, health, and nursing. *Person* refers to the recipient of nursing actions, who may be an individual, a family, a community, or a particular group. *Environment* refers to the recipient's significant others and surroundings, as well as to the setting in which nursing actions occur. *Health* refers to the wellness and/or illness state of the recipient, and *nursing* refers to the actions taken by nurses on behalf of or in conjunction with the recipient.

The connections among the four metaparadigm concepts are clearly made in the following statement: "Nursing studies the wholeness or health of humans, recognizing that humans are in continuous interaction with their environments" (Donaldson & Crowley, 1978, p. 119). This statement may be considered the major proposition of nursing's metaparadigm, reflecting as it does the overall focus of the discipline of nursing. Other propositions state the relationships between and among the metaparadigm concepts and reflect the major areas of interest to the discipline of nursing:

- The principles and laws that govern the life processes, well-being, and optimum functioning of human beings, sick or well
- The patterning of human behavior in interaction with the environment in normal life events and critical life situations
- The processes by which positive changes in health status are effected (Donaldson & Crowley, 1978; Gortner, 1980)

CONCEPTUAL MODELS

The second, and still quite abstract and general, component of the structural hierarchy of nursing knowledge is the conceptual model. The term *conceptual model,* and synonymous terms, such as *conceptual framework, conceptual system, paradigm,* and *disciplinary matrix,* refer to global ideas about the individuals, groups, situations, and events of interest to a discipline. Conceptual models are made up of abstract and general concepts and of propositions that state something about the concepts in an abstract and general manner. An example of a conceptual model concept is *adaptation*, a concept that can refer to all types of individuals and groups, in a wide variety of situations. An example of a conceptual model proposition is "People are rational beings." Another example is "Nursing intervention is directed toward management of environmental stressors."

Uses of Conceptual Models

A conceptual model provides a distinctive frame of reference for its adherents, telling them what to look at and speculate about. Most importantly, a conceptual model determines how the world is viewed and what aspects of that world are to be taken into account. For example, one conceptual model may focus on interventions designed to help a person adapt to stressors, and another may emphasize a person's capacity for self-care.

THEORIES

The third component of the structural hierarchy of knowledge is the theory. A theory may be defined as "a statement that purports to account for or characterize some phenomenon" (Barnum, 1990, p. 1). Theories, like conceptual models, are made up of concepts and propositions. Theories, however, address phenomena with much greater specificity than do conceptual models.

The specificity of a theory requires that its concepts be more specific and concrete than those of a conceptual model. Therefore, they are tied more closely to particular individuals, groups, situations, or events. Examples of such concepts are temperature, pulse, blood pressure, distress, and social support. The propositions of a theory also are more specific than those of a conceptual model. An example is "There is a phenomenon known as social support." Another example is "Social support is defined as supportive transactions that include expression of positive affect of one person toward another; affirmation of another's behavior, perceptions, or views; and provision of symbolic or material aid to another." Still another example is "Social support is positively related to well-being."

68   THE PLACE OF INQUIRY

METAPARADIGMS, CONCEPTUAL MODELS, AND THEORIES

Most disciplines have a single metaparadigm but multiple conceptual models. These are derived from the metaparadigm and, therefore, incorporate the most global concepts and propositions in a more restrictive, yet still abstract manner. Each conceptual model provides a different view of the metaparadigm concepts. The multiple conceptual models of each discipline specify the metaparadigm phenomena in diverse ways. Theories provide still greater specification of these phenomena. Theories are derived from or linked with conceptual models, as Reese and Overton (1970) explained:

> Any theory presupposes a more general model according to which the theoretical concepts are formulated. At the more general levels, the concepts are generally less explicitly formulated, but they nonetheless necessarily determine the concepts at the lower levels. (p. 117)

The abstract nature of conceptual models requires many theories to fully describe, explain, and predict phenomena within the domain of the model. Thus, the structural hierarchy of knowledge progresses from a single metaparadigm to multiple conceptual models and multiple theories derived from each model.

PHILOSOPHY AND SCIENCE

Philosophy may be defined as a statement of beliefs and values about the world, a perspective on human beings and their world, and an approach to development of knowledge (Seaver & Cartwright, 1977). The metaparadigm of a discipline identifies the phenomena about which philosophic statements are made. Conceptual models and the theories derived from them reflect those philosophic statements.

Conceptual models of nursing, like the conceptual models of other disciplines, reflect different philosophic beliefs about the nature of person-environment relationships. For example, Roy's adaptation model of nursing is based on philosophic assumptions that encompass several values and beliefs associated with the general principles of humanism and veritivity. Humanism, according to Roy (1988), refers to "a broad movement in philosophy and psychology that recognizes the person and subjective dimensions of human experience as central to knowing and valuing" (p. 29). The tenets of humanism that are relevant to Roy's conceptual model are based in the notions of creative power, purposefulness, holism, subjectivity, and interpersonal relations. Roy believes that the individual "(a) shares in creative power, (b) behaves purposefully, not in a sequence of cause and effect, (c) possesses intrinsic holism, and (d) strives to maintain integrity and to realize the need for relationships" (p. 32). *Veritivity* is a philosophical premise that asserts that "there is an absolute truth" (p. 29). As a principle of human nature, veritivity "affirms a common purposefulness of human existence" (p. 30). Roy believes that "the individual in society is viewed in the context of the (a) purposefulness of human existence, (b) unity of purpose of humankind, (c) activity and creativity for the common good, and (d) value and meaning of life" (p. 32).

Science may be defined as the systematic, controlled, empirical, and critical activities undertaken to generate and test theories (Kerlinger, 1986). Metaparadigms are not science per se, but rather identify the phenomena to which scientific activity is directed in a discipline. Conceptual models also are not science, inasmuch as the abstract and general nature of conceptual model concepts and propositions precludes direct empirical observation or test. Theories also are not science but are, at least in the case of empirical theories (Carper, 1978), the product of science. Thus science, as defined here, stands outside the structural hierarchy of knowledge as an empirical endeavor.

CONCLUSION

My answer to the question posed must be that contemporary conceptualizations of nursing, in the form of our metaparadigm, conceptual models, and theories, are neither philosophy *nor* science. Rather, philosophy guides the focus of conceptual models and science produces theories, the contents of which are derived from conceptual models.

REFERENCES

Barnum, B. J. S. (1990). *Nursing theory. Analysis, application, evaluation* (3rd ed.). Glenview, IL: Scott, Foresman/Little, Brown Higher Education.

Carper, B. A. (1978). Fundamental patterns of knowing in nursing. *Advances in Nursing Science, 1*(1), 13-23.

Donaldson, S. K., & Crowley, D. M. (1978). The discipline of nursing. *Nursing Outlook, 26,* 113-120.

Eckberg, D. L., & Hill, L., Jr. (1979). The paradigm concept and sociology: A critical review. *American Sociology Review, 44,* 925-937.

Gortner, S. R. (1980). Nursing science in transition. *Nursing Research, 29,* 180-183.

Kerlinger, F. N. (1986). *Foundations of behavioral research* (3rd ed.). New York: Holt, Rinehart & Winston.

Kuhn, T. S. (1977). Second thoughts on paradigms. In F. Suppe (Ed.), *The structure of scientific theories* (2nd ed., pp. 459-517). Chicago: University of Illinois Press.

Reese, H. W., & Overton, W. F. (1970). Models of development and theories of development. In L. R. Goulet & P. B. Baltes (Eds.), *Life span developmental psychology. Research and theory* (pp. 115-145). New York: Academic Press.

Roy, C. (1988). An explication of the philosophical assumptions of the Roy Adaptation Model. *Nursing Science Quarterly, 1,* 26-34.

Seaver, J. W., & Cartwright, C. A. (1977). A pluralistic foundation for training early childhood professionals. *Curriculum Inquiry, 7,* 305-329.

7

Philosophical Inquiry in Nursing: An Application

✳

BARBARA A. CARPER

The concept of *knowledge* is not a topic with which we are ordinarily preoccupied in the conduct of our everyday affairs. The ordinary notion of knowledge seems to have a definite, easily comprehensible, and commonly shared meaning. However, if each of us were asked to respond thoughtfully to such questions as, "What do I know?", "How do I come to know what I know?", "What counts for me as evidence?", and "What criteria do I use to determine the truth?", we would, sooner or later, conclude that we have "different ways of constructing reality, different definitions of what was real and unreal, sensible and nonsensical, during the course of any one day" (Leshan & Margenau, 1982, p. 9). On further reflection, we would also conclude that each of our different constructions of reality, in terms of what we know and how we come to know it, makes sense to us. In fact, we might say that it is common sense that we do *not* know everything in the same way. "Yet to ask ourselves these questions and to reflect on our answers is more than an intellectual exercise," as Belenky, Clinchy, Goldberger, and Torule (1986) make clear:

For our basic assumptions about the nature of truth and reality and the origins of knowledge shape the way we see the world and ourselves as participants in it. They affect our definitions of ourselves, the way we interact with others, our public and private personae, our sense of control over life events, our views of teaching and learning, and our conceptions of morality. (p. 3)

The importance of these questions concerning the nature of knowledge and of reality extends beyond the concerns of each of us as individuals into the issues and debates surrounding knowledge development and utilization for nursing. At the time I first asked myself what kinds of knowledge a nurse requires, I was concerned, not only from the perspective of a nurse educator, as to what we should teach. My question also had its origin in my experiences and perspective as a clinician. There seemed to be a lack of coherence between what I was teaching and how I actually practiced nursing. For me, at that time, the teaching and the practice of nursing were separate, although related, realities. These very personal and pragmatic concerns were the genesis of my study (Carper, 1975) that identified what I called the "fundamental patterns of knowing in nursing."

FUNDAMENTAL PATTERNS OF KNOWING IN NURSING

Purposes

The primary purposes of the study were to (a) utilize a systematic approach for the analysis of selected nursing literature that would serve to identify the structure of knowledge in nursing, and (b) identify the fundamental patterns of knowing that characterize and exemplify the discipline of nursing.

Method of Analysis

Inquiry into the nature of knowledge belongs in the field of epistemology, that branch of philosophy concerned with the study of human knowledge. Therefore, the approach selected for inquiry into the structure of knowledge and patterns of knowing in nursing was a systematic and critical analysis of the nursing literature from a philosophic point of view. The aim of inquiry in this study was not to extend the range of what is known. The purpose was, rather, to engage in disciplined, critical reflection, following logical rules, to achieve a clearer understanding of the kinds of knowledge comprising the discipline of nursing.

Criteria for Selection of Literature

Literature selected for analysis was restricted to nursing textbooks and journals, not specified for or limited to a specialty area of nursing, published within the 10-year period of 1964-65 to 1974-75.

Sequence of Analysis

The systematic analysis of selected nursing literature was based on the logical-conceptual-methodological model developed by Phenix (1964). The purpose of this model is to describe the distinctive logical types of knowledge as identified by their representative ideas or concepts and their modes of inquiry or methods of discovery and verification. The sequence of the analysis was guided by the following questions:

1. What is the substantive/conceptual structure of knowledge in nursing?
   a. What are the representative concepts that specify, describe, define, and/or classify the phenomena of the discipline of nursing?
   b. What constructs and/or dominant themes indicate how these representative concepts are related to each other in a systematic way?
   c. What concepts and/or conceptual models are characteristic in that they direct or control inquiry in the discipline?
2. What is the syntactical structure of knowledge in nursing?
   a. What are the methods of inquiry?
   b. What methods are used to validate/test claims to knowledge?
   c. What methods of inquiry exhibit the patterns of explanation and/or prediction?

FINDINGS

The Substantive/Conceptual Structure

Representative Concepts. Those concepts identified as representative of the phenomena most relevant, important, and meaningful to nursing as a discipline were man, health, patient-client, nursing, and behavior. *Man* was described (almost without exception in the selected literature) in terms of his integrated biopsychosocial wholeness. The interest and concern of the discipline of nursing in man was conceived to be regulated and determined by the specific dimension of his health. *Health* was characterized as a relative state or fluctuating level of wellness rather than by a discrete either/or concept. The concept of *patient-client* identified an individual as a recipient of nursing care by virtue of his location on the health-illness continuum. *Nursing* was conceptualized as a deliberate, goal-directed, action-oriented process that cannot be defined apart from the recipient of nursing care. The purposes and goals of nursing were variously described as assisting, helping, providing, supporting, promoting, enabling, and facilitating the patient-client in such a way that health is maintained, illness prevented, or recovery facilitated. The nature of problems presented by patient-clients requiring nursing action were primarily conceptualized in terms of *behavior* or *behavioral responses.*

Conceptual Models. The concepts of man, health, patient-client, nursing, and behavior—the representative ideas of nursing— specify the phenomena of interest and carry direct implications for defining the subject matter of the discipline. The several conceptual models described in the literature elaborated how these concepts may be related to each other in a systematic way and how they could or should function as guides for inquiry in the development of knowledge for the discipline.

Each of these conceptual models utilized the representative concepts, as well as a variety of other related concepts, to describe the relevant variables affecting or influencing man's behavior, his state of health, his status as a patient-client, and the purpose or goal of nursing action. However, each of the models defined these concepts in different ways so that the meaning of the conceptual terms and the assumed or postulated relationships among them, the terminology employed, and the explication of the related variables cannot be understood apart from the context of the particular model. Each of these models suggested different kinds of problems to be solved and varied in regard to what factors or events were considered to be most relevant or important. The possibility that each might lead eventually to dissimilar bodies of knowledge and different goals of nursing action could not be ignored.

The Syntactical Structure

The second component of the structure of knowledge has to do with the methods of inquiry for the discovery and verification of knowledge. The nursing literature clearly identified the primary methods of inquiry to be theory development and empirical (scientific) research. Theory development, as a method of inquiry, had a variety of meanings which were reflected in two identifiable divergent orientations to the generation and verification of theoretical knowledge. The two divergent approaches, one based on the inductive model, the other on the deductive, were widely debated in the literature in terms of how they influence the generation of nursing science.

Those who subscribed to the inductive approach to theory development tended to emphasize that the area of actual nursing practice should constitute the phenomenological field for the observation and collection of empirical data, which eventually would lead to inductively formulated empirical generalizations and scientific theory. Others proposed that a priori construction of a theoretical reality, from which propositional or hypothetical statements were derived and then verified or falsified by empirical evidence, was more congruent with the traditional method of "doing science."

In addition to the scientific methodology for the development and validation of a theoretical and empirical body of knowledge, there was also a clearly identifiable method of inquiry for the *practice* of nursing, the nursing process. It was a fundamental and pervasive method in that it was applicable in any setting and to any of the various conceptual structures.

The nursing process, as a method of inquiry, involves a complex and diverse combination of methodological activities that require different kinds of observations and evidence, different kinds of explanations, and different kinds of reasoning. The process involves a multistep and goal-oriented series of inferences and judgments in which the selection and interpretation of information is colored by value considerations and moral issues for which scientific, theoretical knowledge is necessary, but not sufficient, for understanding.

Fundamental Patterns of Knowing

Four fundamental patterns of knowing in nursing were identified as a result of the analysis of the substantive/conceptual and syntactical structures of knowledge. Each of the four fundamental patterns was distinguished according to the logical type of meaning and were designated as (a) *empirics*, the science of nursing; (b) *ethics*, the component of moral knowledge; (c) *personal knowledge*; and (d) *esthetics*, the art of nursing.

Empirics: The Science of Nursing. The empirical pattern of knowing in nursing is concerned with matters of fact that are expressed in descriptions or in statements of relationship between phenomena that are asserted to be true or probable. Empirical data, obtained by either direct or indirect observation and measurement, if verified through repeated testing over time, are formulated as scientific principles, generalizations, laws, and theories that provide explanation and prediction. Scientific knowledge is objective, abstract, and general. Quantifiability of data allows objective measurement, which yields evidence that is capable of replication by multiple observers and is therefore publicly verifiable.

Ethics: The Moral Component. The moral dimension of nursing is concerned with choosing, justifying, and judging action. It involves the notions of moral duty and obligation. Ethical choice requires rational and deliberate reasoning. Ethical knowledge is normative and abstract as well as singular and particular. Moral choice is personal in that decisions are voluntary and deliberate and the moral agent is held accountable for the judgment made and the action taken. Ethical judgments are particular in that choices and actions occur in concrete situations. But they are also abstract and general in that the moral rules or principles that justify the action taken are held to be universally valid and generalizable to all similar situations. Moral actions are not simply a function of personal values but are informed and mediated by

membership in the moral community of nursing. Ethical knowledge also involves the examination and evaluation of what is
good, valuable, and desirable as ends or goals, motives, and traits
of character.

Personal Knowledge. This pattern of knowing is concerned with
knowledge of self and self in relation to others. Self-consciousness
permits us to know ourselves and other selves unmediated by conceptual categories or particulars abstracted from complex wholes.
Personal knowledge is necessarily subjective, concrete, and existential and does not require mediation through language. It does require engagement rather than detachment, and an active, empathic
participation of the knower.

Esthetics: The Art of Nursing. This pattern of knowing is knowledge of that which is individual, particular, and unique. Esthetic
knowledge requires the active transformation of what is observed,
through the experience of subjective acquaintance, into a direct,
nonmediated perception of significant relationships and wholes
rather than separate, discrete parts. Esthetic knowledge is the
comprehension and creation of value and meaning from both gen-
eralized abstractions and concrete particulars. It enables us to "go
beyond" what can be explained by existing principles and theories
and to account for variables that cannot be systematically related
or quantitatively formulated. It is interpretive, contextual, intuitive, and subjective knowledge. It requires synthesis rather than
analysis.

DISCUSSION

Although the patterns of knowing have been described as separate and logically distinct ways of knowing, they are not mutually
exclusive. There are multiple points of contact between and among
these patterns of knowing. They are not only interrelated but inter-
dependent. Such interdependence more accurately reflects the complexity and richness of nursing practice and the kinds of knowledge
required in making clinical judgments.

There can no longer be serious doubt that nursing requires different ways of knowing and different kinds of knowledge. The question now is, "How do we support and enable the continuing

development of the kinds of knowledge needed to adequately reflect and accommodate the epistemological plurality of nursing?"

A Model for the Creation, Expression, and Assessment of the Patterns of Knowing

Jacobs-Kramer and Chinn (1988)[1] have recently developed a model that extends each of the patterns by considering how the knowledge is generated, transmitted, and evaluated. The model consists of three dimensions: the creative, the expressive, and the assessment.

The creative dimension is concerned with how knowledge is generated, extended, or modified through use and implies process-product interaction. "To consider the creative dimension is to consider what the knowledge pattern is useful for, and how . . . knowing and knowledge is extended and modified" (Jacobs-Kramer & Chinn, 1988, p. 131). The expressive dimension is conceptualized as the means of recognizing and exhibiting the knowledge in each pattern. The third dimension of the model, assessment, provides for examination of the separate knowledge forms by (a) asking critical questions that assess the adequacy of the knowledge pattern, (b) identifying a process context that is specific to knowledge generation in each pattern, and (c) denoting a pattern-specific credibility index.

The following summarizes the three dimensions of this model for each of the four patterns of knowing:

1. Empirical knowledge is created through the familiar research methodologies for describing, explaining, and predicting. The product, empirical (scientific) knowledge is expressed as facts, models, theories, and descriptions that provide understanding. Empirical knowledge is assessed by asking the critical questions, "What does this represent?" and "How is it representative?" The process and context for addressing these questions is replication. Validity is the index of credibility.

2. The creative dimension of ethical knowledge involves valuing, clarifying, and advocating, which are also the processes for extending knowledge. Ethical knowledge is expressed through codes, moral rules, and decision making. The critical questions asked of ethical knowledge for assessment are, "Is this right?" and "Is this just?" ("Is this good?"). The process context for asking these questions is dialogue and the credibility index is justness.

3. The creative dimension of personal knowledge involves encountering, focusing on, and realizing self and others. Personal knowledge is expressed as an authentic and disclosed self. Assessment involves examining the expression form—the self—for congruity of the authentic self with the disclosed self ("I-Me" congruity). Critical questions—"Do I know what I do?" and "Do I do what I know?"—occur in the process of response and reflection for addressing the credibility index of congruity.

4. The creative dimension of esthetics involves engaging, interpreting, and envisioning, which are also the processes for extending knowledge in this pattern. Esthetic knowledge finds expression in the *art-act*. The knowledge expressed in the art-act is assessed by criticism that is directed toward the interpretation of meaning. The critical question asked is "What does this mean?", and credibility is discerned by reaching consensus.

For each of the patterns of knowing, there are appropriate methods of inquiry for discovery and generation of new knowledge or for the extension, modification, and revision of existing knowledge. Forms for representing or expressing knowledge vary from one pattern to another, as do the criteria for credibility and the critical questions for assessing the value and utility of the knowledge.

CONCLUSION

Nursing is both an academic discipline and a practice profession (Visintainer, 1986). The perspective of nursing, as a practice profession, is critical in both the creation and evaluation of a body of knowledge. The practice of nursing requires not only "knowing that" but also "knowing how" and "knowing why" in regard to meaning, value, intentions, and goals. Benner's (1984) study of clinical nursing practice provides a vivid and compelling description of the complexity and kinds of knowledge used by expert nurses in actual practice. Schultz and Meleis' (1988) reflection on nursing epistemology led them to specify three types of knowledge required for nursing: clinical, conceptual, and empirical. Whatever descriptive categories are employed, the significance of what is being expressed by these nurse scholars and researchers lies in the recognition and acknowledgment that the kinds of

knowledge and the methods of inquiry necessary for the practice
of nursing extend beyond the boundaries of science.

NOTE

1. Used by with permission of Springer Publishing Company, Inc., New York,
10012, from "Perspectives on Knowing: A Model of Nursing Knowledge" by M.
Jacobs-Kramer and P. Chinn, *Scholarly Inquiry for Nursing Practice*, 2(2). Copyright © 1988 by Springer Publishing Company.

REFERENCES

Belenky, J. F., Clinchy, B. M., Goldberger, N. R., & Torule, J. M. (1986). *Women's ways
of knowing.* New York: Basic Books.
Benner, P. (1984). *From novice to expert: Excellence and power in clinical nursing practice.*
Menlo Park, CA: Addison-Wesley.
Carper, B. A. (1975). *Fundamental patterns of knowing in nursing.* Unpublished doc-
toral dissertation, Teachers College, Columbia University.
Jacobs-Kramer, M. K., & Chinn, P. L. (1988). Perspectives on knowing: A model of
nursing knowledge. *Scholarly Inquiry for Nursing Practice, 2*, 129-139.
Leshan, L., & Margenau, H. (1982). *Einstein's space and Van Gogh's sky.* New York:
Collier.
Phenix, P. H. (1964). *Realms of meaning.* New York: McGraw-Hill.
Schultz, P. R., & Meleis, A. I. (1988). Nursing epistemology: Traditions, insights,
questions. *Image, 20*, 217-221.
Visintainer, M. A. (1986). The nature of knowledge and theory in nursing. *Image, 18*,
32-38.

PART THREE

The Future of
Philosophic Inquiry in Nursing

Will the time come when the scope of nursing research courses includes philosophic nursing research? When philosophic inquiry is accepted as being integral in the same degree as scientific inquiry to the realm of nursing research? When nurses recognize which nursing questions they are asking are philosophic and which are scientific and, in turn, use the appropriate mode of inquiry to answer each kind of question?

Are nurses, today, willing to supply philosophic nursing inquiry with the kind of nourishment it requires to flourish? Or will they continue to feed nursing science almost exclusively to the detriment of the profession? The essays by Fry (Chapter 8) and Schlotfeldt (Chapter 9) in Part Three provide ample motivation for nurses to consider the future of philosophic inquiry in nursing.

Both essays are suggestive of some conditions that must be met if philosophic inquiry is to make its much needed contribution to nursing knowledge development in the future. The question arises: What other conditions are required? Can philosophic inquiry in nursing develop and progress in the face of unshared notions or definitions of philosophy or must one of the conditions be that nursing embrace a common definition?

At the outset of her essay, Fry points out that she is about to add still another definition of philosophy to those already put forward by other authors. This problem of definition brings us full circle to reconsider what was said in Part One. There, several different definitions of philosophic inquiry are operative, each reflecting a different philosophic position on the nature of reality and of knowledge. In some cases, the position taken is explicitly revealed; in others, not. This is also true of the essays in Part Two and is a state of affairs that characterizes the nursing literature at large.

Until nurses begin to address this definitional problem, the future of philosophic inquiry in nursing is apt to remain a mystery. It is crucial that nursing authors not leave the presuppositions underlying their philosophic positions unstated. They must be made explicit and available for discussion. Only under those conditions do we stand a chance of arriving at the truth of the matter with regard to the nature of philosophic inquiry in nursing, its potential usefulness, and its future in nursing knowledge development. The sound advancement of nursing as a profession will, in large part, be determined by whether or not philosophic inquiry in nursing in fact becomes a nursing activity with a future. In turn, this depends (in part) on how we answer questions such as those that follow.

Guiding Questions: Making Up Your Own Mind

1. Is the neglect of philosophical inquiry in nursing apparent or real?

2. On what basis ought we to decide whose responsibility it is to answer philosophic questions about nursing matters?

3. What does deciding philosophic nursing matters on the basis of consensus presuppose?

4. Is it necessary that answers to nursing's philosophic questions be agreed upon by adherents of the discipline? If not, by what means can the discipline progress? If so, in what manner or by what means can agreement be soundly attained?

5. What conditions (philosophical, social, political, and economic) are required for philosophic inquiry to flourish in nursing?

6. What are the implications for the future of nursing as a profession of coming, or of not coming, to understand the nature of philosophic inquiry in nursing and of identifying its place in our nursing research endeavors?

8

Neglect of Philosophical Inquiry in Nursing: Cause and Effect

*

SARA T. FRY

INTRODUCTION

I would like to express my thanks to June Kikuchi, Helen Simmons, and the rest of the nursing faculty at the University of Alberta for hosting this conference and for inviting so many stimulating and interesting people to attend. The exchange of thought has been very worthwhile and I predict that it will be helpful to the development of nursing thought and inquiry, as well. June and Helen are to be commended for sharing their thoughts so willingly and for their receptiveness to the thoughts and ideas of others. I am sure that I speak for everyone when I say that I wish you well in the development of the Institute for Philosophical Nursing Research and many more conferences of this nature.

CAUSE AND EFFECT PHENOMENA

I have been asked to address the topic of the cause and effect of the neglect of philosophical inquiry in nursing. The title of this topic presupposes, of course, that philosophical inquiry in nursing has, in fact, been neglected and that the cause and effect of that neglect can be delineated—clearly pinpointed, named, and/or described.

First, I would like to point out that I am not convinced that philosophical inquiry has been intentionally neglected in nursing. I am of the opinion that nurses have been asking philosophical questions about the nature of the nurse/patient relationship, the interactions between ill individuals and their environments, and the moral foundations of nursing practice, since the time of Nightingale. In addition, several of our early nurse leaders conducted rather thorough examinations of topics of interest to nursing using philosophical methods of inquiry. The reason that they asked certain questions and pursued them with philosophical methods of inquiry is that they were well-educated women. Any well-educated person prior to World War II studied philosophy and was expected to use philosophy in the way that he/she looked at the world and discussed human affairs.

Nursing, however, in attempting to build its research and theoretical bases, has favored scientific inquiry over other forms of inquiry. Schools of nursing on academic campuses aligned nursing inquiry with scientific inquiry in an earnest desire to have nursing command respect in the academic environment. As a result, beginning with the 1940s and continuing to the present time, philosophical inquiry has simply taken a back seat to scientific inquiry in nursing. As graduate education in nursing flourished, we encouraged a whole generation of nurse researchers and nurse educators to value scientific inquiry as opposed to other forms of inquiry. Our theory development literature amply documents this fact (Andreoli & Thompson, 1977; Benoliel, 1977; Ellis, 1968; Jacox, 1974; Johnson, 1959). The brave souls who did engage in philosophical inquiry were not recognized and, as Barbara Carper points out (Chapter 7), they found it difficult to get their works published. Control of the journals is one way that any developing discipline defines and shapes the preferred style of thought of the discipline (Fleck, 1935/1979; Toulmin, 1972).

My point is that the so-called neglect of philosophical inquiry is really a devaluation of philosophical inquiry or a failure to recognize such inquiry for what it is. The effects of this devaluation and nonrecognition are made manifest in the following:

- A lack of funding for philosophical studies
- Student resistance to the study of philosophical methods or reluctance to undertake philosophical inquiry

• Few nurses knowledgeable about philosophical inquiry in the profession as a whole, but especially among those responsible for nursing education

Despite these effects, philosophical inquiry enjoys a rather interesting role in nursing at the present time. Its role has been shaped by our historical traditions as well as by our conceptions of nursing as a human science that is primarily empirically defined. Although I do not particularly want to defend any of these ideas—they stem from intuition more than anything else and are stated as opinion rather than fact—I do think I can identify where philosophical inquiry is taking place in nursing; offer some ideas about the state-of-the-art of philosophical inquiry; and, finally, suggest some future directions that might be pursued in order to strengthen and broaden the multiple uses of philosophy in nursing. If we can be satisfied with this more temperate treatment of the topic of "neglect of philosophical inquiry in nursing," then it is probably safe to proceed.

DEFINING PHILOSOPHICAL INQUIRY

In this book, several definitions of the term *philosophy* have been provided. Two of these are (a) a set of beliefs about the world, and (b) a mode of inquiry to answer certain questions. To confuse matters, I will give one more definition by stating that philosophy is the study of the universe at large and the world of human affairs. To philosophize or to *do* philosophy is to raise questions, make and defend arguments, and bring systematic reflection to bear upon our ideas about our experience, the universe, and human affairs. Two goals of such philosophizing would be to discover and understand (a) how the universe is constructed, and (b) how humans live or ought to live (Hamlyn, 1970). There are probably other goals of philosophy but, for now, these will suffice.

Is philosophy the special realm or expertise of only those who are academically prepared in philosophy? I do not think so. In fact, it seems that every well-educated person uses and does philosophy to a greater or lesser degree. Hence, apologies for not being a philosopher or not being educationally prepared to function as a philosopher do not excuse anyone from doing philosophy. There is no special magic associated with academic preparation in philosophy. All such preparation really provides is the expectation that those so educationally prepared are expected to do *more* philosophy than someone who is not similarly prepared. Philosophers are expected to function primarily as philosophers rather than in some other way.

For example, asking philosophical questions is something that everyone does. Knowing when certain questions are best answered by philosophical methods of inquiry is something that we should all recognize. Carrying out philosophical inquiry, however, requires knowledge about philosophical methods and how to employ them. Although philosophical questioning and argumentation can be undertaken by just about anyone, it seems that extended philosophical investigation requires more than everyday knowledge about philosophy. Such investigations tend to be done by philosophers, but they can be done by others, as well.

With these reflections about the nature of philosophical inquiry in mind, let me now note the areas in which philosophical inquiry is taking place in nursing. Although there are probably many such areas, three come to mind: (a) the feminist critique of science, (b) nursing epistemology, and (c) nursing ethics. Because of the time limitation, I will only discuss the second area—nursing epistemology.

NURSING EPISTEMOLOGY

In general, traditional epistemology has centered on three questions, questions that have been or are currently being asked in nursing:

1. What can be known or believed to be true?
2. What counts as criteria for the objects of knowledge?
3. How can one assert knowledge of himself/herself or knowledge of others?

With respect to the first question—"What can be known or believed to be true?"—several directions of thought within nursing are apparent. One direction assumes that nursing knowledge is unique and asserts the existence of research questions, methodologies, and topics that are called "nursing" rather than something else. An example of this approach is the attempt to define and delineate the consensus on nursing functions as established by research (Haller, Reynolds, & Horsley, 1979). A second direction assumes that knowledge is borrowed and adopts the pragmatic application of theories, frameworks, and experimental manipulation of interventions in order to explain, predict, or control nursing phenomena. The use of life stress models, taken primarily from psychology, to explain behavior and establish the relationship of multiple variables as predictors of health outcomes is an example of this direction (Flaskerud & Halloran, 1980).

The second question—"What counts as the criteria for the objects of knowledge?"—has been taken up in many works that address the nature of science in nursing, the perspective of the applied scientist in nursing, and the nature of nursing science. These works have addressed empirical qualities of nurse/patient states, physiological measures of patients, measurable aspects of health states, and anything that can be empirically defined and on which numerical data can be obtained. Most of this research has followed Carper's (1978) notion of the science of empirics and the use of empirical methodologies to explain, control, and predict nursing phenomena.

Although some work has been done in an effort to define the moral phenomena of nursing practice, work in this area is still at a very early stage of development. Likewise, little work has been done in the areas of aesthetic knowledge, the art of nursing, and personal knowing. Questions concerning these patterns of knowing have not been framed in a manner that allows for systematic study or that yields empirical data. The one exception to this research pattern is the growing amount of discussion and scholarship in nursing devoted to the caring phenomenon (Griffin, 1983; Leininger, 1981, 1984; Ray, 1984; Watson, 1985).

Caring is being described as a human phenomenon that requires empirical knowing, ethical knowing, and, possibly, personal knowing for the explication of its richness and diversity. Given the current interest in caring as a central value of nursing, we might see a great deal of research devoted to nurse caring in the years ahead.

With regard to the third and last epistemological question— "How does one assert knowledge of the self and knowledge of others?"—I do believe that a considerable amount of work in nursing has addressed this type of question. Phenomenological investigations of empathy, grief, the reaching-out experience, the mental states and experiences of individuals in significant life events, as well as the bereavement process have all been undertaken in different contexts and with different populations (Andre, 1985; Parse, 1985). Studies of this type often address the mental states of the investigator as well as those of others, with the purpose of explicating the essence of the state or the experience.

Given the development of these types of studies and the questions that have been asked, I conclude that the nature of knowledge for nursing, in terms of traditional questions about knowledge, have been and will continue to be addressed in nursing. However, work of this nature often goes unrecognized for what it is. Either the nature of the question in relation to nursing science is not prominent or there is a failure to recognize the research question as basically philosophical in nature. If either is the case, what might be suggested as a unifying theme for philosophical investigations in nursing and their relevance to the various forms of nursing knowledge?

PHILOSOPHY OF NURSING

One of the problems to be avoided in any attempt to unify the development of nursing knowledge is the placement of the forms of nursing knowledge within a structure that limits inquiry. Carper (1978) addresses patterns of knowing within a well-defined structure that is ultimately related to nursing practice and change. Her structure allows for adjustment of the patterns of knowing according to new information from the practice realm and changing thought. Donaldson and Crowley (1978), on the other hand, lock the development of nursing knowledge into predetermined categories as defined by the perspective of nursing. They view the nursing perspective as an absolute standard that is unchanging over time and as necessary to the discipline of nursing.

Considering the current state of knowledge development in nursing, we might want to seriously question the tendency to predetermine categories of acceptable thought in nursing. Why should nursing inquiry—philosophical or otherwise—be characterized as possessing an identifiable structure that can be delineated and articulated *prior* to the explication of that knowledge or the outcomes of inquiry? Why would this be desirable given the early stage of nursing's theorizing and the recognized need to avoid closure on the forms of nursing inquiry at the present time (Suppe, 1982)? Unfortunately, nursing seems to have a long history of using this approach to theorizing. We have consistently borrowed conceptual and theoretical frameworks from other disciplines, borrowed other forms of inquiry, and adopted criteria for the evaluation of theorizing. We have then attempted to structure our own theorizing within these borrowed frameworks. Why is there this tendency in nursing? Do we need to do this where nursing epistemology is concerned? Perhaps we should even ask: What other alternatives are there?

Fortunately, there are a few alternatives to the formalized structures of inquiry currently being proposed for nursing. In fact, there are good reasons why one should *not* attempt to articulate the structures of inquiry prior to knowing the outcomes of inquiry. According to some philosophers in contemporary epistemology, it is prudent to resist the structuring of knowledge development in any form. Rorty (1979), for example, in his critique of epistemology since Descartes, strongly argues against the structure of inquiry, especially against the attempt to do epistemology that mirrors or represents the world in terms of identifiable structures. Indeed, many contemporary scholars across the humanities and the sciences are moving toward the "deconstruction" of inquiry and are "dismantling" the structures of knowledge that have constrained and confined the limits of human inquiry within their respective disciplines (Culler, 1982; Derrida, 1982; Gadamer, 1975; Guba & Lincoln, 1982; Norris, 1982, 1985). Building on the works of Heidegger (1927), Dewey (1929), Wittgenstein (1953), Kuhn (1970), and contemporary continental philosophy (Gadamer, 1975, 1981), the humanities and the social sciences are giving serious attention to the problems inherent in the "structure of the discipline" emphasis that permeated education and the social sciences in the 1950s and 1960s. Many are moving away from this emphasis and toward recognition of the social construction of knowledge or are simply recognizing the need to define knowledge apart from a priori categories of thought.

Nursing, however, still under the influence of curriculum development needs, has not seriously considered other approaches to articulating the nature of inquiry until just recently. Doctoral programs in nursing are beginning to include course content on the philosophy of science and discussion of contemporary reactions, within both the sciences and the humanities, to the "received view on theory." However, despite this content, many nurse scholars have difficulty incorporating what should be learned from philosophy in terms of the analysis and understanding of our own theorizing. It seems that nurse scholars are simply hesitant to engage in the necessary "self-consciousness" (to use the terminology of Dr. Jan Thompson, 1985) to formulate the questions that need to be answered as well as to clearly articulate the modes of nursing inquiry that might be utilized to answer those questions.

Fortunately, inquiry in nursing is in an early stage of development. No theories of nursing pursuing particular types of questions have been widely accepted and nursing inquiry is not strongly formalized within any structure of inquiry at the present time. Given this stage of knowledge development within nursing, what might be proposed for the future development of nursing science?

I propose that we locate nursing science and nursing inquiry within an understanding of a philosophy of nursing (Fry, 1988). If a model of a philosophy of nursing could be proposed, the relationship between the various forms of inquiry important to the development of nursing knowledge might be as portrayed in Figure 8.1.

I show this figure with some reluctance because the depiction of these ideas in the form of a model could easily be interpreted as a proposed structure within which inquiry takes place. My intention is not to do this. Given the arguments that I have just given against a priori structures of inquiry, what I am trying to illustrate is that nursing uses various forms of inquiry, such as epistemology, ethics, and metaphysics, which complement each other and are recognized as important to the development of nursing knowledge. The fact that they are all philosophical forms of inquiry is no accident. If one talks about the process of developing a philosophy of nursing, it is expected that philosophical forms of inquiry will be prominent (Fry, 1988).

I am proposing a philosophical model for the development of nursing science for two reasons: One reason concerns the nature of nursing; the other concerns the nature of philosophy. Both of these reasons deserve some explanation.

First, philosophy is the study of the universe at large and the world of human affairs. Nursing, because it is also concerned about the world of human affairs, is fundamentally a human science.

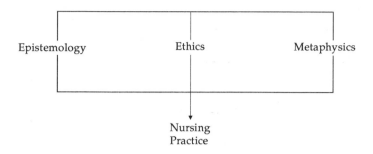

Figure 8.1. A Model of a Philosophy of Nursing

Hence, philosophical inquiry has special meaning for nursing and for the human sciences. It is a form of inquiry that uses critical analysis to explicate and to evaluate information and beliefs. It has already been used in nursing with some success and thus has already found a small but important place within nursing inquiry (Gadow, 1980; Lanara, 1981; Smith, 1983).

Second, philosophy often functions as a heuristic device to uncover the various ways we understand a practice as an applied science and as a practice that incorporates various kinds of concepts as well as facts. Within nursing, philosophy functions as a formal, analytical tool for inquiry—an analytical tool to make explicit the rules of inference that guide reasoning in nursing. Therefore, *doing* the philosophy of nursing includes several related endeavors: (a) analysis and description of the concepts and language of nursing; (b) systematic reflection on nursing theories and the body of nursing knowledge as it addresses human needs; and (c) development of the methodology and metatheory of nursing judgments, including moral judgments.

Ethical inquiry is an essential part of the philosophy of nursing insofar as it (a) describes moral phenomena encountered in the practice of nursing; (b) addresses the basic claims of rights and duties, and goods and values, as they arise within the practice of nursing; and (c) assesses the language of rights and duties,

94 THE FUTURE OF INQUIRY

and of goods and values, as a rational endeavor (Englehardt & Erde, 1980). The roles and forms of inquiry can be recognized in the endeavors of a philosophy of nursing identified earlier. The forms of inquiry complement and are complemented by the elements of epistemology, ethics, and metaphysics of nursing. Using the methods of argumentation commonly utilized in doing philosophy, the forms of inquiry address descriptive, normative, and meta-ethical dimensions of the phenomena of nursing science.

Beyond the methods of argumentation and the forms of inquiry, however, no structure or a priori framework within which inquiry should take place is being proposed. Philosophical inquiry is merely conceptually located within the philosophy of nursing to help move nursing inquiry toward the use of philosophy as a vehicle in attempts to establish the theoretical foundations for research and practice in nursing. When philosophical inquiry is so located, the relationships between the modes of inquiry are readily evident. This will help us to understand how philosophy can be used in nursing and the kinds of questions that a philosophical perspective might address.

In the final analysis, perhaps it is not philosophical inquiry that has been neglected in nursing scholarship, but rather our openness to visualize philosophical inquiry as necessary and fundamentally important with respect to establishing the theoretical foundations of nursing practice and research. It might be appropriate to recognize such inquiry for what it is and to conceptually locate philosophical inquiry within a framework of relevance to the practice of nursing and its social role in society.

REFERENCES

Andre, N. J. (1985). The lived experience of reaching out: A phenomenological investigation. In R. R. Parse (Ed.), Nursing research: Qualitative methods (pp. 119-132). Bowie, MD: Brady Communications.
Andreoli, K. G., & Thompson, D. C. (1977). The nature of science in nursing. Image, 9(2), 32-37.
Benoliel, J. (1977). The interaction between theory and research. Nursing Outlook, 25(2), 108-113.
Carper, B. A. (1978). Fundamental patterns of knowing in nursing. Advances in Nursing Science, 1(1), 13-23.
Culler, J. (1982). On deconstruction: Theory and criticism after structuralism. Ithaca, NY: Cornell University Press.

Derrida, J. (1982). *Margins of philosophy*. Chicago: University of Chicago Press.

Dewey, J. (1929). *The quest for certainty*. New York: Minton, Balch.

Donaldson, S. K., & Crowley, D. M. (1978). The discipline of nursing. *Nursing Outlook, 26*(2), 113-120.

Ellis, R. (1968). Characteristics of significant theories. *Nursing Research, 17*(3), 217-222.

Englehardt, H. T., & Erde, E. L. (1980). Philosophy of medicine. In P. T. Durbin (Ed.), *A guide to the culture of science, technology, and medicine* (pp. 364-461). New York: Free Press.

Flaskerud, J. H., & Halloran, E. J. (1980). Areas of agreement in nursing theory development. *Advances in Nursing Science, 3*(1), 1-7.

Fleck, L. (1979). *Genesis and development of a scientific fact* (T. J. Trenn & R. K. Merton, Eds.; F. Bradley & T. J. Trenn, Trans.). Chicago: University of Chicago Press. (Originally published as *Entstehung und entwicklung: Einer wissenschaften Tatsache*. Basel: Benno Schwabe, 1935)

Fry, S. T. (1988). The nature of knowledge. In C. Bridges & N. Wells (Eds.), *Proceedings of the Fifth Nursing Science Colloquium* (pp. 7-23). Boston: Boston University School of Nursing.

Gadamer, H. G. (1975). *Truth and method* (G. Barden & J. Cumming, Trans.). New York: Seabury Press.

Gadamer, H. G. (1981). *Reason in the age of science* (F. G. Lawrence, Trans.). Cambridge, MA: MIT Press.

Gadow, S. (1980). Existential advocacy: Philosophical foundations of nursing. In S. F. Spiker & S. Gadow (Eds.), *Nursing: Images and ideals* (pp. 79-101). New York: Springer.

Griffin, A. P. (1983). A philosophical analysis of caring in nursing. *Journal of Advanced Nursing, 8*, 289-295.

Guba, E. G., & Lincoln, Y. S. (1982). Epistemological and methodological bases of naturalistic inquiry. *Educational Communication and Technology Journal, 30*, 233-252.

Haller, K. B., Reynolds, M. A., & Horsley, J. A. (1979). Developing research-based innovation protocols: Process, criteria, and issues. *Research in Nursing and Health, 2*, 45-51.

Hamlyn, S. W. (1970). *The theory of knowledge*. London: Macmillan.

Heidegger, M. (1927). *Being and time* (J. Macquarrie & E. Robinson, Trans.). London: SCM Press.

Jacox, A. (1974). Theory construction in nursing: An overview. *Nursing Research, 23*(1), 4-13.

Johnson, D. E. (1959). The nature of a science of nursing. *Nursing Outlook, 7*(5), 291-294.

Kuhn, T. S. (1970). *The structure of scientific revolutions* (2nd ed.). Chicago: University of Chicago Press.

Lanara, V. A. (1981). *Heroism as a nursing value: A philosophical perspective*. Athens: Sisterhood Evniki.

Leininger, M. M. (Ed.). (1981). *Caring: An essential human need. Proceedings of the Three National Caring Conferences*. Thorofare, NJ: Slack.

Leininger, M. M. (1984). *Care: The essence of nursing and health*. Thorofare, NJ: Slack.

Norris, C. (1982). *Deconstruction: Theory and practice*. London: Methuen.

Norris, C. (1985). *Contest of faculties: Philosophy and theory after deconstruction*. London: Methuen.

Parse, R. R. (1985). The lived experience of health: A phenomenological study. In R. R. Parse (Ed.), *Nursing research: Qualitative methods* (pp. 27-37). Bowie, MD: Brady Communications.

Ray, M. A. (1984). The development of a classification system of caring. In M. M. Leininger (Ed.), *Care: The essence of nursing* (pp. 95-112). Thorofare, NJ: Slack.

Rorty, R. (1979). *Philosophy and the mirror of nature.* Princeton, NJ: Princeton University Press.

Smith, J. (1983). *The idea of health: Implications for the nursing professional.* New York: Basic Books.

Suppe, F. (1982). Implications of recent developments in philosophy of science for nursing theory. In *Proceedings of the Fifth Biennial Eastern Conference on Nursing Research* (pp. 10-16). Baltimore: University of Maryland School of Nursing.

Toulmin, S. (1972). *Human understanding* (Vol. 1). Princeton, NJ: Princeton University Press.

Thompson, J. (1985). Practical discourse in nursing: Going beyond empiricism and historicism. *Advances in Nursing Science, 7*(4), 59-71.

Watson, J. (1985). *Nursing: Human science and care.* New York: Appleton-Century-Crofts.

Wittgenstein, L. (1953). *Philosophical investigations* (G. E. M. Anscombe, Trans.). New York: Macmillan.

9

Answering Nursing's Philosophical Questions: Whose Responsibility Is It?

✳

ROZELLA M. SCHLOTFELDT

This chapter provides an answer to one timely and important philosophical question in the field of nursing—that which appears in its title. In this essay, the widely accepted definition of the term *responsibility* as a charge, duty, or obligation; or that for which one is accountable or answerable (*Webster's Third New International Dictionary*, 1976, p. 1935) is adopted. Further, the paper is based upon a major assumption: Nursing, as an institutionalized, beneficially consequential field of service that is essential and sometimes crucial to the health and well-being of all people at particular times during their lives, holds potential for becoming, and is becoming generally recognized as, a primary, learned health profession and academic discipline. Based upon acceptance of the meaning of responsibility and of the assumption stated, the answer to the question posed in the title of this presentation is unequivocal. Scholarly professionals who are nurses hold a responsibility for answering nursing's philosophical questions.

Two reasons justify the response given to the question posed. The first is that societies give to members of each profession, to which they grant positive sanction, the prerogative—indeed the obligation—to identify, explicate, and transmit to its trainees not only the knowledge and expertise needed by its practitioners, but also the values and the moral and ethical code that the profession endorses that is expected to guide the conduct of individuals who are admitted to its membership and permitted to practice (Larson, 1977; Wilensky, 1964). Moreover, societies hold the expectation that all fields of work that qualify as professions will be self-governing and that professionals will monitor practices and censure any among them who fail to demonstrate adherence to the groups' standards of practice, their professional values, and their ethical codes.

The second justification for the response given to the question posed is that none, except those who are practitioners of the nursing profession and who are able, inquiring scholars with the requisite nursing knowledge, clinical nursing experience, interest, and expertise, know and can articulate what nursing's philosophical questions are and can be depended upon to seek and find reliable, satisfactory answers to them.

Surely, the answer given to the question posed, and the logic presented for its justification, can hardly be challenged. Why then, after over a century of nursing's existence as an institutionalized field of essential human service, during which many nursing leaders have aimed and claimed to be preparing professionals, is it necessary to discuss the question of who holds responsibility for answering nursing's philosophical questions? And after more than 3 decades of preparing rapidly increasing numbers of nursing scholars, why have those nursing scholars not already addressed and found acceptable answers to nursing's most important philosophical questions?

It must be recognized that nursing has made quite remarkable progress over the past half century in amassing a large group of well-prepared, competent professionals for the field. And, in the more recent decades, nursing has made quite spectacular gains in preparing a significant number of those professionals as productive, inquiring scholars. Many of them have made significant contributions to knowledge and surely qualify as learned, scholarly professionals. Yet, in 1989, nursing is still considered by many of its critics and by some nurses to be an ambiguous and enigmatic field of work.

Evidence cited to support those allegations includes the fact that nursing leaders have eschewed responsibility for identifying and explicating the differences between and among nursing professionals, technicians, and a host of assisting personnel; leaders in the field have also failed to ensure that recognized differences in competencies of those several kinds of practitioners are reflected in credentialing mechanisms and in the expectations held for them in numerous health care settings.

They observe further that nurses themselves, scholars among them, seem not to be in agreement about what nursing's essential role is nor about what preservice preparation is required for those seeking to become qualified to enter professional practice.

With humility that derives from the speaker's perceived inadequacy to the assigned task, two more philosophical questions are identified to which qualified nursing scholars have not yet found answers on which they can agree. The legitimacy of those questions may be a topic that scholars may wish to consider and to determine how they, and other equally qualified scholars, can find answers upon which they can all agree and how answers to those questions can be kept current. The two questions are (a) what is the nature of nursing; and (b) what is the nature and scope of professional knowledge that is fundamental to the professional practices of general and specialized nursing practitioners, that is, of that knowledge that comprises the nursing discipline.

Nursing scholars' seeming neglect, to date, of answering those questions may be explained by the observation that there may not yet be nursing scholars in sufficient number who are qualified, committed, and able to devote sufficient time to fulfil the profession's need to have that responsibility met. But it must be recognized as well that, to date, no organized group of scholarly professionals in the field, whose collective membership has the necessary expertise, has been charged with or has assumed that responsibility. Indeed, until this date, there probably have been no opportunities for representative groups of scholarly nursing professionals to engage in significant, sustained discussion (and debate) concerning the questions posed with the goal of finding answers to them upon which they can agree. Certainly the University of Alberta's Nursing Faculty members deserve great commendation for their leadership in establishing an Institute for Philosophical Nursing Research, which may serve as a catalyst for providing North American nursing scholars, from academic and clinical settings alike, with such opportunities in the future.

THE NATURE OF NURSING

From the time of nursing's existence as an identifiable occupation, individual nurses have set forth conceptualizations concerning the nature of nursing, beginning with Florence Nightingale (Nightingale, 1859). Early in the 20th century, when nursing leaders sought and attained legal control over nursing practice and the preservice preparation of practitioners as well, nursing was defined in the several jurisdictions' laws. Each of those definitions reflected the influence exerted on legislators, not only by the several state and provincial nurses' organizations, but also by politically powerful individuals and groups of individuals who sought to have maximal control over nurses, nursing practice, and nursing education. That circumstance still prevails, with the consequence that leaders and scholars in nursing have no effective voice in developing the legal definitions that prescribe the nature of nursing. Those definitions are still determined in the political arena, and they reflect all of the extensions, expansions, restrictions, and changes in nurses' responsibilities that are imposed by power brokers, whose influences upon nursing are dominant each time nurse practice laws are opened and changed.

In the mid-20th century, Henderson's (1961) definition of nursing was given widespread acceptance by nurses throughout the world when it was adopted by the International Council of Nurses (p. 42). Since that time, Henderson's definition has seemingly lost favor. Presently, some legal definitions of nursing reflect the current diagnoses and treatment fashion (American Nurses' Association, 1980); others do not.

In the last 2 decades, several individual nurses have set out their conceptualizations of the nature of nursing, often mislabeled *theories* of nursing. All compete for advocates and supporters. Nursing faculties typically vote for their favorite one, which then serves as a conceptual guide or framework for their respective curricula. Nursing staffs of service agencies, too, by vote or mandate select one, from several, to guide their work. Should a philosophical question concerning the nature of nursing be answered by political pressures? By popular vote? By mandate?

Considerable agreement can be found among some of the conceptualizations of nursing that have been put forth by various creative nurses. It is agreed that assisting human beings attain optimal levels of health represents the essence of nursing's goal and practice responsibilities (Fawcett, 1983). But major differences are also evident when one compares and contrasts some of the several definitions and conceptualizations of nursing that currently exist (Schlotfeldt, 1987). Those differences sometimes point to quite disparate phenomena with which nurses are expected to deal in practice and concerning which nursing scholars should be expected to advance knowledge. It appears that the time is overdue for nursing scholars to be given, or to take responsibility for giving, unequivocal answers to the question, "What is the nature of nursing? What approach is needed to ensure attainment of that worthy goal?"

THE DISCIPLINE OF NURSING

The second philosophical question posed in this paper relates to the nature and scope of professional knowledge that comprises the nursing discipline. Finding the answer to that question is crucial because it will identify the content or subject matter that, at any particular time in history, should be mastered and internalized for use by all who seek to have the privilege of engaging in general or specialized practice in the field of professional nursing.

There is quite general agreement that the discipline encompasses knowledge of the history of nursing's development over time, particularly those factors, events, and people whose influences on its status and its emergence toward professionhood have been noteworthy. It includes, as well, philosophical content concerning the profession's values and the moral and ethical principles to which the profession adheres. It includes the profession's scientific knowledge.

NURSING HISTORY

It is of interest that nursing has typically depended upon its own members to document its heritage and development. One reason for that may be that until the recent past, scholars in the general field of history did not consider the history of occupations and professions to be of general historical import. Because nursing leaders perceived nursing's history to be of interest, there was no alternative but to have nurses record it. The consequence was that scholarship in nursing history represented nursing's initial foray into the research enterprise.

Currently, some general historiographers are manifesting interest in the history of all the health professions. Meanwhile, a slowly growing group of nurses have become formally qualified historians engaged in scholarly pursuit of knowledge concerning various aspects of nursing's history. It would appear that, henceforth, nursing's history should be increasingly well documented. Further, the establishment of centers for the study of nursing history in prestigious universities and the existence and visibility of nursing archives should encourage nurses to commit themselves to scholarship in that field.

NURSING PHILOSOPHY

Undoubtedly influenced by authors who set forth criteria that should be fulfilled by occupations in order to merit recognition as professions, nursing leaders called for the development of a code of nursing ethics early in the occupation's existence (*American Journal of Nursing*, 1903). Although debate ensued relevant to the need for such a code, one nurse produced a text on the subject (Robb, 1900) and, in 1921, an advisory committee of nurses was charged with responsibility to develop nursing's ethical code (Viens, 1989).

It has been suggested that nursing's early ethical codes were primarily statements concerning etiquette and morality expected to be demonstrated by nurses (Kelly, 1985, p. 205). Nonetheless, such a code has been in existence since 1940 (Viens, 1989, p. 47); it has served as a guide for nursing practitioners. Organized nursing's insistence on having such a code, however, has not been consistently matched by efforts of nursing faculties to require that philosophical content be prerequisite to, or an integral part of, curriculum requirements for preservice programs of professional nursing education.

In the recent past, a small but steadily growing number of nurses have earned Ph.D. degrees in the discipline of philosophy. It is expected that those scholars will be increasingly depended upon for help to resolve some of the philosophical dilemmas that nurses encounter in executing their practice, teaching, investigating, administering, and policymaking roles and for assistance in finding answers to the more general, unanswered philosophical questions that were presented earlier, as well.

NURSING SCIENCE

Nursing science is surely the largest and most rapidly changing content encompassed in nursing's discipline. Traditionally, nursing depended entirely upon basic and medical scientists to discover all of the science that comprised the scientific aspects of its intellectual armamentarium. Even after nursing's research movement was well under way, little clinical research designed to discover knowledge fundamental to nursing practice was ongoing (Henderson, 1977) and, even now, few investigations guided by nursing theories concerning phenomena of direct interest and concern to practitioners have been undertaken. After the mid-20th century, when nurses in increasing numbers earned research degrees, first in the basic sciences and later in nursing as well, they primarily sought in their scientific inquiries to test the relevance of basic science concepts, propositions, and theories, for application in nursing practice (Chinn, 1984; Silva, 1986).

Considerable rhetoric has been generated and reported in nursing's recent literature about the need for nursing theories and for the identification of phenomena of interest and concern to nurses about which theories should be developed. But few nurses have identified human phenomena that are or should be of theoretical interest to nursing's scholarly practitioners and theorists (Schlotfeldt, 1987). The fact that few nursing scholars are actively involved in, and making decisions about, nursing practice problems (activities that would put them in a position to identify gaps, contradictions, and errors in nursing science) is likely directly relevant to that lack (Schlotfeldt, 1989). Recent calls for nurses' discovery of knowledge that is "imbedded in clinical nursing practice" (Benner, 1984, p. 1) may provide the needed stimulus for scholarly nursing practitioners to become theorists and for theorists to have active involvement in nursing practice—practice that includes decision making and the execution of theory- and science-based, philosophically sound nursing strategies designed to assist human beings to attain reasonable health goals and their health potentials.

SUMMARY

It has been the intent in this essay to provide an unequivocal and reasonable answer to the question of who should take responsibility for answering nursing's philosophical questions. An equally important question to be addressed surely is how nursing's scholarly practitioners can be assured or can assure themselves that they will henceforth have opportunities for adequate, sustained discourse through which to reach agreement in discharging that arduous and important responsibility.

REFERENCES

American Journal of Nursing. (1903). Report of the sixth annual convention of the nurses' associated alumnae of the United States [Entire issue]. *3:* 856.
American Nurses' Association. (1980). *Nursing: A social policy statement.* Kansas City, MO: Author.
Benner, P. (1984). *From novice to expert.* Menlo Park, CA: Addison-Wesley.
Chinn, P. (1984). From the editor. *Advances in Nursing Science, 6*(2), ix.
Fawcett, J. (1983). Hallmarks of success in nursing theory development. In P. Chinn (Ed.), *Advances in nursing theory development* (pp. 3-17). Rockville, MD: Aspen.
Henderson, V. (1961). *Basic principles of nursing care.* London: International Council of Nurses.
Henderson, V. (1977). We've come a long way, but what of the direction? [Guest Editorial] *Nursing Research, 26*(3), 163-164.
Kelly, L. Y. (1985). *Dimensions of professional nursing* (5th ed.). New York: Macmillan.
Larson, M. (1977). *The rise of professionalism: A sociological analysis.* Berkeley: University of California Press.
Nightingale, F. (1859). *Notes on nursing: What it is and what it is not.* London: Harison, 59, Pall Mall.
Robb, I. H. (1900). *Nursing ethics for hospital and private use.* Cleveland: Koeckert.
Schlotfeldt, R. (1987). Defining nursing: A historic controversy. *Nursing Research, 36*(1), 64-67.
Schlotfeldt, R. (1989). The scholarly nursing practitioner. In C. A. Lindeman (Ed.)., *Alternate conceptions of work and society: Implications for professional nursing* (pp. 15-29). Washington, DC: American Association of Colleges of Nursing.
Silva, M. (1986). Research testing nursing theory: State of the art. *Advances in Nursing Science, 9*(1), 1-11.
Viens, D. C. (1989). A history of nursing's code of ethics. *Nursing Outlook, 37*(1), 45-49.
Webster's Third New International Dictionary. (1976). Springfield, MA: Merriam.
Wilensky, H. (1964). The professionalization of everyone? *American Journal of Sociology, 70*(3), 137-141.

Epilogue: Getting to the Heart of the Matter

❋

In the preceding essays, we have been presented with an array of philosophical positions held by scholars in nursing on some major contemporary philosophical nursing issues. These issues have arisen as a result of recent developments in nursing—most notably, our decreasing preoccupation with research methods per se and our increasing preoccupation with theory development.

That philosophic inquiry in nursing is in its infancy is a fact to which the essays in this volume attest. The potential that lies within philosophic inquiry to disclose and anchor nursing's natural (legitimate) power to benefit society and to become a relatively autonomous discipline (i.e., autonomous in relation to other disciplines) has yet to be realized. It is our contention that this potential will remain unrealized unless and until the central philosophic nursing issues, within which the issues raised in the separate essays in this volume are subsumed, are resolved. Given that the advancement of nursing as a learned profession in part depends on the successful resolution of such issues, it is fitting to consider what this resolution requires of us.

We must come to grips with what the nature of philosophic inquiry in nursing is, what its place in nursing inquiry is, and what its future can and must be. In getting on with this formidable task, we are faced with conditions in nursing that constitute both the best of times and the worst of times for the undertaking. As we know, nursing, in its efforts to become fully professionalized and recognized as such, has been beset with problems: some, a result of a lack of awareness of its distinction from other disciplines; some due to its inappropriate tendency to emulate the behavioral and social sciences.

In effect, it has conducted itself according to prevailing fashion, allowing itself to be controlled by outside influences rather than engaging in sustained philosophic study of what constitutes its own distinctiveness.

Although, in the past, individual nurses have philosophized about the nature of nursing, it is only very recently that the profession, disillusioned with science and burdened with the consequences of the technologies science it has spawned, has formally begun to seek answers to some of its philosophic questions. However, the search has been episodic and largely limited to questions of an ethical and epistemological nature, to critical/analytical aspects of the philosophic endeavour, and to the phenomenological, hermeneutic, and existential approaches of continental philosophy.

In this move by nursing toward formal philosophizing, another special problem is emerging: the adopting of a particular philosophic school of thought in the absence of an adequate understanding of the suppositions, the presuppositions, and the implications inherent in the position adopted. The inherent danger is that nursing has made itself vulnerable to being contradictory in its assertions and to erroneously using the scientific mode of inquiry in instances where the philosophic mode ought to be used.

An accompanying problem, also just beginning to show itself in the nursing literature, is the use of philosophic jargon that cannot be understood by those who are not adherents of the particular school of thought from whence the jargon springs. As a consequence, it is difficult, and at times impossible, to come to terms with authors, which considerably decreases the common understanding required for pleasurable and profitable philosophic dialogue. This latter problem is especially foreboding in light of three very recent, encouraging developments in nursing.

The first of those encouraging developments is that interest in dialoguing about philosophic nursing issues, as opposed to merely listening to "experts'" opinions on such issues, is growing. This desire on the part of nurses to actively engage in philosophic discussion may very well be a function of the fact that an increasing number of nurses are becoming prepared in the area of theory development in nursing, and some even in philosophy. The second is that not only are nursing journals appearing that foster dialogue specifically on the development of nursing knowledge, but also nursing conference planners are no longer entirely eschewing conceptual papers in favour of reports of scientific findings. The third development is that nurse researchers are beginning to acknowledge and use modes of inquiry other than the scientific mode: a development that promises to help meet the need in nursing for knowledge relevant to nursing practice.

Although there are substantial obstacles in the way of our getting on with the work of resolving the philosophic nursing issues requiring our immediate attention, on balance, the conditions to proceed and succeed appear to be better than they have ever been. In addition to generally taking advantage of whatever positive conditions prevail, if we are to succeed, we must get beyond our cherished practice of talking only to the adherents of our preferred school of thought. We must engage those holding opposing positions to see wherein the truth lies with regard to the claims each of us has made. In order to do that, we must abandon the popular stance of taking issue with those with whom we differ and join together to get to the heart of the matter before us. This means that we must examine those assumptions and presuppositions we are holding to be true that give rise to our differences and that in an enlightened state we might not hold. The key to getting to the heart of any matter is to ask questions of each other that are likely to reveal our assumptions and presuppositions—a difficult but essential and achievable activity, as Plato so clearly demonstrated 2500 years ago.

Undertaking the kind of actions just described, will, in the doing, essentially shape a community of nursing scholars, scholars invested in bringing to fruition, through sustained disciplined dialogue, the potential that sits in philosophic nursing inquiry for the sound advancement of the profession.

—June F. Kikuchi
—Helen Simmons

Index

✳

About the Editors

✳

June F. Kikuchi, R.N., Ph.D., holds the positions of Professor and Director of the Institute for Philosophical Nursing Research (IPNR) at the University of Alberta, Faculty of Nursing, Edmonton, Alberta, Canada. She received a B.Sc.N. from the University of Toronto, and an M.N. and a Ph.D. (in Nursing Care of Children) from the University of Pittsburgh. Postdoctorally, she studied Philosophy at the University of Toronto. She is the co-founder of the IPNR. She has published papers on philosophic nursing inquiry and knowledge, nursing knowledge development, and the quality of life of children of disabled parents. She has presented papers nationally and internationally on those topics as well as on the development of nursing research in health care agencies. She is the co-organizer of a series of biennial invitational philosophic nursing conferences, "Philosophy in the Nurse's World."

Helen Simmons, Ph.D., holds a joint appointment as Special Projects Consultant at the Edmonton Board of Health Nursing Division, and as Associate Professor and Associate Director of the Institute for Philosophical Nursing Research (IPNR) at the University of Alberta, Faculty of Nursing, Edmonton, Alberta, Canada. She received a B.A. (Psychology and Philosophy) and an M.A. (Clinical Psychology) from the

University of British Columbia, and a Ph.D. (Educational Psychology) from the University of Oregon. She has pursued studies in Philosophy, postdoctorally, at the Aspen Institute for Humanistic Studies. She is the co-founder of the IPNR and is the co-organizer of the "Philosophy in the Nurse's World" conference series. Her publications and presentations have focused on health, public health, philosophic nursing inquiry and knowledge, and nursing knowledge development. She was awarded an honorary life membership in the Alberta Association of Registered Nurses for her contributions to the nursing profession.

About the Contributors

✳

Evelyn Adam, R.N., M.N., holds the position of Professor Emeritus at the University of Montreal, Faculty of Nursing, Montreal, Quebec, Canada. She received a Diploma in Nursing from the Hôtel-Dieu Hospital in Kingston, Ontario, a B.Sc.N. from the University of Montreal, and an M.N. from the University of California at Los Angeles. Her articles about conceptual models for nursing and her book, *To Be a Nurse*, which is published in four other languages as well, are frequently cited in the nursing literature by students and scholars. Through her independent consultant practice, she continues to make available her expertise in the development and application of conceptual models for nursing.

Barbara A. Carper, R.N., Ed.D., F.A.A.N., is the Interim Dean, College of Nursing, University of North Carolina at Charlotte, Charlotte, North Carolina. She is a baccalaureate graduate of Texas Woman's University and received an M.Ed. and an Ed.D. from Teachers College, Columbia University. Postdoctorally, she studied in Medical Ethics at Harvard University as a Visiting Scholar. Her particular area of interest is the analysis and development of nursing theory and the ethical dimensions of nursing. Her seminal work on the "Fundamental Patterns of

Knowing in Nursing" has served and continues to serve nurses well in their scholarly endeavors.

Jacqueline Fawcett, R.N., Ph.D., F.A.A.N., is a Professor at the University of Pennsylvania, School of Nursing, Philadelphia, Pennsylvania. She holds a B.S. (Nursing) from Boston University and an A.M. (Parent-Child Nursing) and a Ph.D. (Nursing) from New York University. She is the author of the well-known and widely used text, *Analysis and Evaluation of Conceptual Models of Nursing* (now in its second edition) and is co-author of the book, *The Relationship of Theory and Research.* She is the author of several articles and book chapters dealing with the nature of nursing knowledge, and is author or co-author of several research reports in the area of maternity nursing.

Sara T. Fry, R.N., Ph.D., F.A.A.N., is an Associate Professor at the University of Maryland, School of Nursing, Baltimore, Maryland. She received a Diploma (Nursing) from the Johns Hopkins School of Nursing, a B.S. (Nursing) from the University of South Carolina at Columbia, an M.S. (Public Health Nursing) from the University of North Carolina at Chapel Hill, and an M.A. (Philosophy) and a Ph.D. (Philosophy) from Georgetown University. She was a Kennedy Fellow in Medical Ethics at Georgetown University from 1981 to 1982, and a Visiting Scholar at the Kennedy Institute of Ethics, 1990 to 1991. She is the co-author of the book, *Case Studies in Nursing Ethics* (1987). She has published widely and presented numerous papers nationally and internationally on the topics of bioethics, the ethics of health care technologies, and professional ethics. She has received several honors and awards for her work in bioethics.

John R. Phillips, R.N., Ph.D., is an Associate Professor at the New York University, Division of Nursing, New York, New York. He holds a Diploma (Nursing) from the Bellevue Schools of Nursing, a B.S.N. from Hunter College—Bellevue School of Nursing, and an M.A. (Nursing) and a Ph.D. (Nursing) from New York University. He has presented and published several papers in the area of nursing knowledge development, most notably and recently in the journal, *Nursing Science Quarterly* for which he serves as an editorial board member.

Sister M. Simone Roach, R.N., Ph.D., is the CSM/Board Liaison at St. John's Hospital, Lowell, Massachusetts. She received a B.Sc.N. from St. Francis Xavier University, an M.S. (Administration Nursing Education) from Boston University, and a Ph.D. (Foundations of Education-Philosophy) from The Catholic University of America. She was a postdoctoral Visiting Scholar in Ethics at the Harvard Divinity School from 1980 to 1981. She has worked primarily in nursing education in Canada and, in philosophy, in the area of caring. Her publications, *Caring: The Human Mode of Being* and *The Human Act of Caring: Blueprint for the Health Professions,* have received recognition nationally and internationally.

Rozella M. Schlotfeldt, R.N., Ph.D., F.A.A.N., holds the position of Professor Emeritus and Dean Emeritus at the Case Western Reserve University, School of Nursing, Cleveland, Ohio. She received a B.S. (Nursing) from the University of Iowa, and a S.M. (Nursing Education/Administration) and a Ph.D. (Education Curriculum Development) from the University of Chicago. She holds seven honorary doctoral degrees as well as many other significant awards. She is recognized and respected nationally and internationally for her substantial contributions to the development of the nursing profession, particularly in the area of nursing education and of nursing knowledge development. She has presented papers widely and published extensively in books and in professional nursing journals and newsletters. She has served on numerous occasions as a visiting professor and has held a wide variety of prominent offices within nursing organizations.